CARDIOVASCULAR
RISK FACTORS

**A Slide Atlas of Cardiovascular
Risk Factors,** based on the
material in this book, is available.
The collection consists of
numbered 35mm slides of each
illustration in the book. The
material is presented in an attractive
binder, which also contains a copy
of the book. The Slide Atlas is
available from:

Gower Medical Publishing,
Middlesex House,
34-42 Cleveland Street,
London WIP 5FB

Gower Medical Publishing
101 5th Avenue, New York,
NY 10003, USA

CARDIOVASCULAR RISK FACTORS

John D Swales MA, MD, FRCP
Professor of Medicine
Leicester University Medical School
Leicester, UK

David P de Bono MA, MD, FRCP
British Heart Foundation Professor of
Cardiology (University of Leicester)
Glenfield General Hospital, Leicester.
Honorary Consultant Cardiologist
Groby Road General Hospital
Leicester, UK

Gower Medical Publishing • London • New York

Distributed in USA and Canada by:
Raven Press Ltd.
1185 Avenue of the Americas
New York
New York 10036
USA

Distributed in rest of the world by:
Gower Medical Publishing
Middlesex House
34-42 Cleveland Street
London WIP 5FB
UK

Publisher:	Michele Campbell
Project Manager:	Richard French
Design:	Louise Bond
Illustration:	Lee Smith
Index:	Anne McCarthy
Production:	Susan Bishop

British Library Cataloguing in Publication Data:
Library of Congress Cataloging in Publication Data:
Catalogue records for this title are available

ISBN 1-56375-551-3

Originated in Hong Kong by Mandarin Offset (H. K.) Ltd.

Produced by Mandarin Offset (H.K.) Ltd.

Printed and bound in Hong Kong

Text set in Granjon; figures and legends set in Gill Sans by
M to N Typesetters, London

PREFACE

One of the most predictable consequences of medical advance has been the escalation of the costs of health care. This and the well established belief that prevention is better than cure has led to a growing interest in preventive medicine. This is a field where clinical medicine, epidemiology and laboratory research all have a great deal to contribute. We have, in the present book, integrated existing knowledge of risk factors for cardiovascular disease. Whilst we have laid strong emphasis on management, we have endeavoured to define the underlying scientific principles and evidence upon which management is based. This is a topic which is particularly suited to illustration and we are indebted to Gower Medical Publishing for producing so much illustrative material for us and to the authors of the following Gower books for some of the illustrations: Diabetes (J Bodansky), Lipids and Lipid Disorders (MD Feher and W Richmond), Hyperlipidaemia in Practice (DJ Galton and W Krone) and Clinical Atlas of Hypertension (JD Swales, PS Sever and WS Peart).

DP de Bono
JD Swales

ADDENDUM

In Chapter 1, Figures 1.6, 1.7 and 1.9 are reproduced from *Clinical Atlas of Hypertension* by Professor J D Swales, Professor P S Sever and Professor W S Peart (Gower Medical Publishing, 1991).

In Chapter 3, Figures 3.1 - 3.11, 3.13 - 3.20, 3.23 - 3.28 and 3.31 are reproduced from *Clinical Atlas of Hypertension* by Professor J D Swales, Professor P S Sever and Professor W S Peart (Gower Medical Publishing, 1991).

In Chapter 4, Figures 4.1 - 4.9, 4.11, 4.13 - 4.19, 4.22 - 4.25, 4.26a, 4.26b - 4.31 and 4.33 - 4.36 are reproduced from *PPG Lipids and Lipid Disorders* by Dr M D Feher and Dr W Richmond (Gower Medical Publishing, 1991). Figures 4.10, 4.12, 4.20, 4.21, 4.32 and 4.37 are reproduced from *Hyperlipidaemia in Practice* by Professor D J Galton and Professor W Krone (Gower Medical Publishing, 1991).

In Chapter 5, Figures 5.1, 5.15 - 5.20, 5.22 - 5.26 and 5.29 - 5.31 are reproduced from
PPG Diabetes by Dr J Bodansky (Gower Medical Publishing, 1989).

In Chapter 6, Figure 6.3 is reproduced from *Clinical Atlas of Hypertension* by Professor J D Swales, Professor P S Sever and Professor W S Peart (Gower Medical Publishing, 1991).

In Chapter 10, Figures 10.10, 10.12 and 10.14 - 10.16 are reproduced from *Clinical Atlas of Hypertension* by Professor J D Swales, Professor P S Sever and Professor W S Peart (Gower Medical Publishing, 1991).

In Chapter 11, Figures 11.2 and 11.4 are reproduced from *Clinical Atlas of Hypertension* by Professor J D Swales, Professor P S Sever and Professor W S Peart (Gower Medical Publishing, 1991).

CONTENTS

Introduction   1

INCIDENCE

Cardiovascular disease is the commonest cause of death, in the middle-aged and elderly, in most Western societies. This is partly due to a decline in other previously important causes of death, such as infectious disease (Figs 1.1 & 1.2). Despite the increased proportionate importance of cardiovascular disease in recent times, in most Westernized countries there has been a decline in cardiovascular deaths. This decline has been particularly marked in the United States and Australia but less evident in the United Kingdom. Thus, the death rate from coronary heart disease has fallen by 19% in men and by 15% in women since 1970 (Fig. 1.3). There has been a steeper decline in strokes which have fallen by more than 30% in both sexes (Fig. 1.4).

Only a small part of the decline in cardiovascular disease is due to the development of new forms of medical or surgical treatment (Fig. 1.5). A much more important contribution has been made by changes in lifestyle, resulting in a reduction in cigarette smoking and serum cholesterol, and by treatment of high blood pressure.

RISK

Risk is a measure of the likelihood of an event occurring. Relative risk can be expressed as a ratio in which the probability of an individual dying from cardiovascular disease is compared to the population average, so that a ratio of 1.3 represents a 30% increase in risk. From the individual's point of view, however, much more important is the absolute risk. For instance, if a patient with high blood pressure has a risk ratio of 2.0 for stroke, this may be fairly unimportant for him if the risk is increased from say 1 in 40,000 to 1 in 20,000. If, on the other hand, the risk of a stroke is increased from 1 in 20 to 1 in 10, this becomes of much more importance.

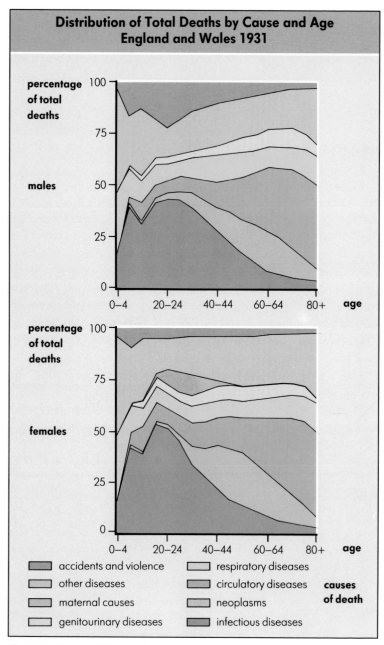

Fig. 1.1 Causes of death in England and Wales in 1931. (Modified from *Health of the Nation*, HMSO 1991.)

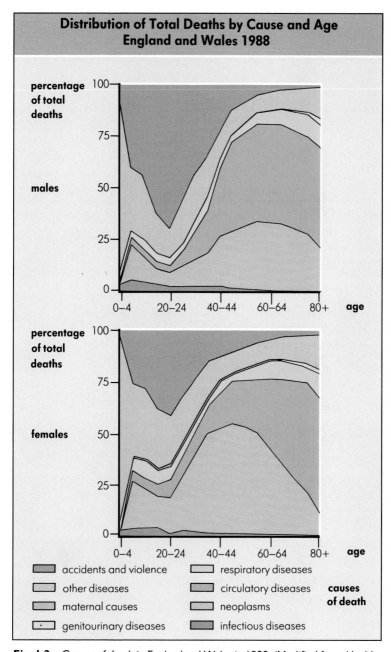

Fig. 1.2 Causes of death in England and Wales in 1988. (Modified from *Health of the Nation*, HMSO 1991.)

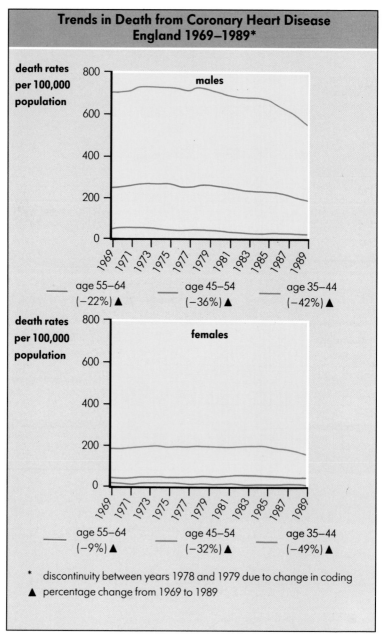

Fig. 1.3 Trends in death from coronary heart disease in England, from 1969 to 1989, in men and women. (Modified from *Health of the Nation*, HMSO 1991.)

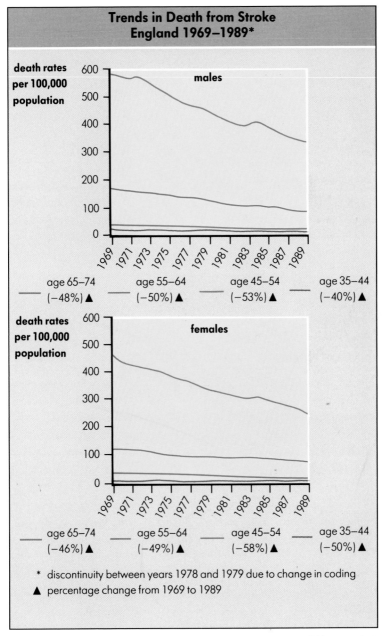

Fig. 1.4 Trends in death from stroke in England, from 1969 to 1989. (Modified from *Health of the Nation*, HMSO 1991.)

5

Estimated Effectiveness of Interventions on Ischaemic Heart Disease Mortality Rates		
	Estimated lives saved	Estimated decline in mortality
Medical interventions	n	%
Coronary care units	85 000	13.5
Prehospital resuscitation and care	25 000	4.0
Coronary artery bypass surgery	23 000	3.5
Medical treatment of clinical ischaemic heart disease	61 000	10.0
Treatment of hypertension	55 000	8.5
Total	249 000	39.5
Changes in lifestyle		
Reduction in serum cholesterol levels	190 000	30.0
Reduction in cigarette smoking	150 000	24.0
Total	340 000	54.0
Not explained or due to errors in preceding estimates	41 000	6.5
Total lives saved	630 000	100.0

Fig. 1.5 Analysis of the contribution of medical interventions and changes in lifestyle, to the overall decline in mortality rates from ischaemic heart disease, in the United States between 1968 and 1976. Most of the decline was due to prevention of ischaemic heart disease rather than management of established ischaemic heart disease. (Modified from Goldman L and Cook EF *Ann Intern Med* 1984; **101**: 825–836.)

Sometimes relative risk and absolute risk can move in opposite directions. For instance the relative risk of hypertension in the elderly is less than in younger age groups. On the other hand, since cardiovascular disease (whether related to hypertension or not) is much more common in the elderly, the absolute risk associated with hypertension is increased (Fig. 1.6).

Identifying individuals at high risk demands that we follow up large numbers of subjects to find out who subsequently develops cardiovascular disease. These data have come from two sources. Life insurance statistics

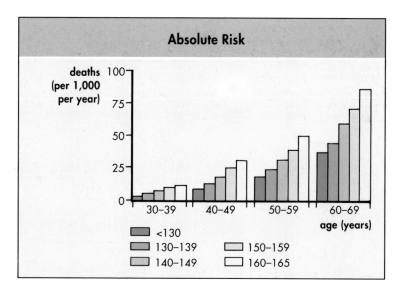

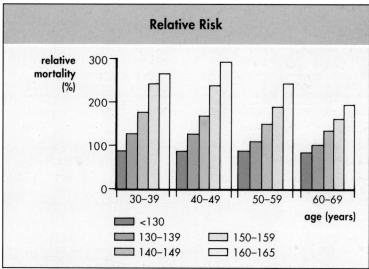

Fig. 1.6 Absolute and relative risk associated with high blood pressure. Note that the relative risk of systolic hypertension in elderly subjects is less than it is in younger individuals. Nevertheless, the absolute risk is much higher since death from cardiovascular disease is much more common in elderly, than in younger individuals (absolute risk equals relative risk multiplied by incidence). (Modified from Rose (1980) *The Hypertensive Patient*. Edited by Marshall & Barritt. London: Pitman Medical.)

provide information on life expectancy in large populations, although the information is very limited. Longitudinal epidemiological investigations (such as the Framingham Study, which has followed up over 5,000 subjects for more than 30 years) have studied smaller populations more intensively. These studies have shown that certain factors in otherwise healthy individuals are associated with an increased risk of subsequently developing cardiovascular disease. This is the 'attributable risk', i.e. the risk attributed to a particular factor (Fig. 1.7).

These factors, therefore, establish individual prognosis. Their value in management depends upon whether they are causally related to cardio-vascular disease or not. Thus, when risk factors, such as high cholesterol or cigarette smoking, are eliminated the risks of cardiovascular disease are at least partially reduced. Other clinical features, such as arcus senilis or transverse ear crease, also identify individuals at increased risk, but even if these could be corrected it would not influence prognosis at all. These are, therefore, 'markers' of risk.

Risk factors can also be classified into those which are reversible, such as smoking, and those which are irreversible, such as age, sex and family background. The distinction between the two may not be sharp. Thus, blood pressure or hyperlipidaemia have both a genetic component and a reversible component which may respond to diet or drugs.

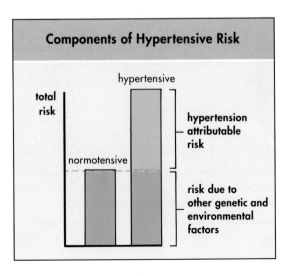

Fig. 1.7 There are two components in the risk of cardio-vascular disease. The excess risk (hypertension attributable risk) and the risk due to other genetic and environmental factors, shared with normotensive subjects.

RISK FACTORS – OVERVIEW

The risk factors identified in the Framingham Study are shown in Fig. 1.8. Although the increase in relative risk may be two or three fold, the absolute individual risk may still be very low, particularly in younger

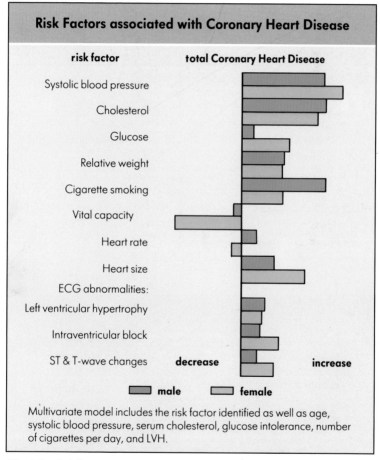

Fig. 1.8   Risk factors associated with development of coronary heart disease in the 30 year follow-up of subjects aged 35 to 64 years in the Framingham Study. Risk is expressed as a standardized logistic coefficient, i.e. the relationship between risk factor severity and the likelihood of subsequent coronary heart disease. (Modified from Stokes J et al. Circulation 1987; v-65–v-73.)

individuals. It is possible to improve on measures of absolute risk by taking several risk factors into account (Fig. 1.9). Mathematical modelling of risk factors suggests that they interact in a multiplicative way so that the presence of several important risk factors such as elevated cholesterol, hypertension and cigarette smoking identifies individuals at high absolute risk (Fig. 1.10). This underlines the importance of screening for several risk factors rather than concentrating on one.

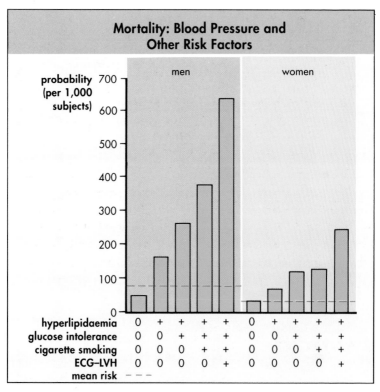

Fig. 1.9 18 year follow-up data from the Framingham Study for patients with systolic hypertension. The presence of other risk factors, such as hyperlipidaemia, glucose intolerance, cigarette smoking or electrocardiographic left ventricular hypertrophy, is associated with a much greater probability of developing cardiovascular disease. (Modified from Kannel & Kreger (1981) in *Blood Pressure Measurement and Systemic Hypertension*. Edited by Arntzenius *et al.* Medical World Publishing.)

Risk Factor Interaction and Death from Cardiovascular Disease in White Men aged 46–57 Years				
Mortality per 1,000				
Group	DBP <90mmHg*	DBP ≥90mmHg	Relative risk†	Excess risk‡
Non-smokers				
Cholesterol <250mg/dl	19.3	25.8	1.3	6.5
Cholesterol ≥250mg/dl	25.4	37.9	1.5	12.5
Smokers				
Cholesterol <250mg/dl	38.8	56.4	1.5	17.6
Cholesterol ≥250mg/dl	50.6	70.7	1.4	20.1

* Results are reported by diastolic blood pressure (DBP), smoking status, and serum cholesterol levels (n = 5,368 deaths).

† Relative risk of mortality in those with DBP ≥90mmHg compared with those with DBP <90mmHg.

‡ Absolute increase in mortality (per 1,000) associated with DBP ≥90mmHg.

Fig. 1.10   Interaction of elevated cholesterol, smoking and diastolic hypertension in risk of death from cardiovascular disease. These three risk factors act in a multiplicative fashion so that an individual with all three risk factors is at very substantially increased absolute risk. (Modified from Browner WS and Hulley SB, Supplement I *Hypertension* 1989; **13**: I-51–I-56.)

STRATEGIES

There are two basic approaches in dealing with risk factors. Population advice is directed at those factors which can be dealt with by changes in lifestyle without the need to identify high risk individuals. Campaigns to reduce smoking and dietary advice to prevent obesity are two examples of this. In other cases strategies may concentrate upon high risk individuals. These can only be identified by population screening. Hypertension and glucose intolerance are cases in point. In other cases both approaches may be adopted as in the case of serum lipids.

Ethnic and Genetic Factors   2

INTRODUCTION

A recurrent theme throughout this book will be that the risk of heart disease in a given individual or community reflects the interplay between genetic susceptibility to disease and environmental factors such as diet, physical exercise, ambient temperature, and smoking habits.

Coronary heart disease has traditionally been regarded as a prerogative of affluent 'Western' communities, but recent epidemiological studies indicate that the incidence of new cases of heart disease is actually falling fastest in the United States, Australia and Northern Europe, and rising most rapidly in newly affluent countries of the 'Third World' and Eastern Europe (Fig. 2.1).

ENVIRONMENT

One of the most striking demonstrations of the interaction between genetics and environment is provided in Neuberger's study of a group of Yemeni Jews who had lived for many centuries at subsistence level in Arabia but were then transported to Israel and provided with a much higher standard of living. The cardiovascular mortality of this group increased dramatically in the first few years after their arrival in Israel, presumably because genetic factors which had been advantageous, or at least harmless, under conditions of severely restricted food intake, became harmful when food intake was increased.

This factor has to be taken into account when comparing cardio-vascular risk in different ethnic groups. A low prevalence of cardiac disease may indicate either a reduced susceptibility, or an environment which does not encourage disease to develop. As a general rule, the prevalence of heart disease in immigrant communities tends to be inter-mediate between the community that they have emigrated from and the

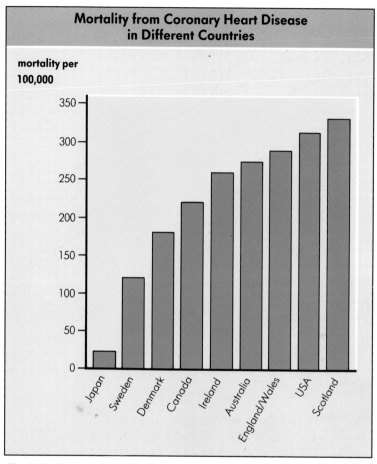

Fig. 2.1 Comparative rates of mortality from ischaemic heart disease in different countries for men aged 45–54 years.

community that they have emigrated into, but there are many exceptions. Cardiovascular disease patterns in major ethnic groups in the United Kingdom are summarized in Fig. 2.2.

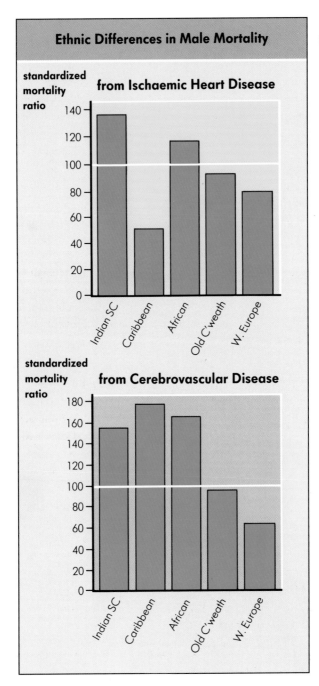

Fig. 2.2 Standardized mortality rates for ischaemic heart disease and cerebro-vascular disease in different ethnic groups in England and Wales from 1979 to 1983. (Modified from Balarajan R *Br Med J* 1991; **302**: 560–563.)

ETHNIC PRESENTATION

The presentation of coronary disease may also vary from community to community. In the United Kingdom, South Asians tend to be over-represented among patients discharged from Coronary Care Units but under-represented among patients with angina referred to cardiology clinics (Fig. 2.3). This may reflect differences in the natural history of the disease, but could also be due to ethnic differences in the appreciation of cardiac symptoms, or to referral bias.

Truly genetic, as opposed to ethnic, influences on coronary risk will be discussed in following chapters, particularly that on lipids. As a general rule, most of the genetic factors which have a major impact on population susceptibility to coronary disease have a relatively small impact on individual life expectancy, and vice versa. For example, familial hyper-cholesterolaemia, which occurs in its heterozygous form in approximately 1 in 500 of the population, has a major impact on the coronary disease risk of sufferers, yet accounts for less than 2% of the population burden of coronary heart disease. This is because, in population terms, patients with

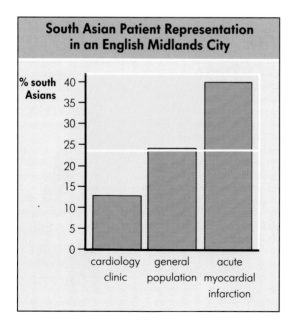

Fig. 2.3 Odds ratios for South Asians in Leicester, England, compared to the rest of the population for: a) Referrals to a cardiology unit with suspected ischaemic heart disease; and b) Hospital discharges after acute myocardial infarction.

familial hypercholesterolaemia are actually very rare, although their individual risk is high. If the total prevalence of coronary disease in the population were to be reduced, the relative importance of conditions, such as familial hypercholesterolaemia, would progressively increase.

EPIDEMIOLOGICAL FACTORS

Within communities, changes in major risk factors such as smoking, total plasma cholesterol concentration and incidence of diabetes tends to have similar relative effects on cardiovascular disease risk even though mean values may vary markedly from community to community and the absolute prevalence of coronary disease may differ (Fig. 2.4). It is important to appreciate this when devising screening, or primary prevention strategies, which involve making decisions based on absolute measurements, such as total plasma cholesterol. An appropriate action level for one community may be totally inappropriate when applied to another.

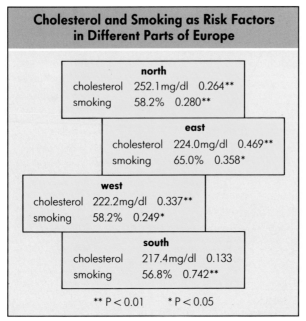

Cholesterol and Smoking as Risk Factors in Different Parts of Europe

north		
cholesterol	252.1mg/dl	0.264**
smoking	58.2%	0.280**

east		
cholesterol	224.0mg/dl	0.469**
smoking	65.0%	0.358*

west		
cholesterol	222.2mg/dl	0.337**
smoking	58.2%	0.249*

south		
cholesterol	217.4mg/dl	0.133
smoking	56.8%	0.742**

** P < 0.01   * P < 0.05

Fig. 2.4 Effects of cholesterol concentration and percentage of total population smoking on ischaemic heart disease mortality in communities from North, West, East and South Europe. (Modified from ERICA research group *Eur Heart J* 1991; **12**: 291–297.)

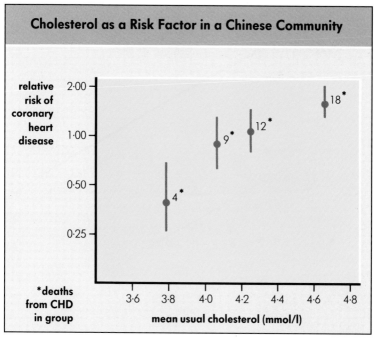

Fig. 2.5 Relationship between cholesterol concentration and cardiovascular mortality in a Chinese community with a low mean population cholesterol concentration and a low prevalence of coronary artery disease. (Modified from Chen Z et al. Br Med J 1991; **303**: 276–282.)

The results in Fig. 2.4 are expressed as multiple logistic regression coefficients, which can be regarded as a measure of the strength of the link between the observed effect (cardiovascular death) and the suggested cause. Thus, the larger the number, the stronger the link. Note that the correlation is positive for smoking in all regions, and for cholesterol in all regions except the South (Italy).

Sometimes it can be interesting to learn from ethnic groups which have a very low prevalence of ischaemic heart disease. In China, where ischaemic heart disease is uncommon and mean population cholesterol levels very low, there is nevertheless still a strong positive correlation between cholesterol concentration and cardiovascular risk (Fig. 2.5). Conversely, there is no evidence from these communities that a very low plasma cholesterol increases the risk of death from other causes.

Hypertension as a Risk Factor   *3*

EPIDEMIOLOGY

Systolic and diastolic blood pressures are distributed as smooth unimodal curves. Any dividing lines between 'hypertensive' and 'normotensive'

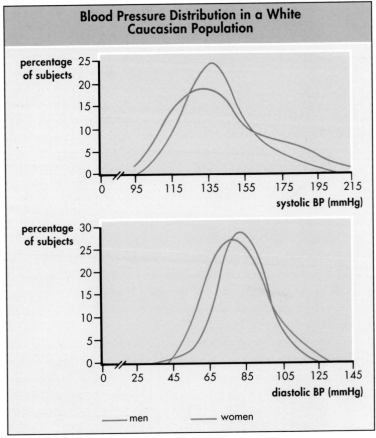

Fig. 3.1   Systolic and diastolic Caucasian blood pressure distribution.

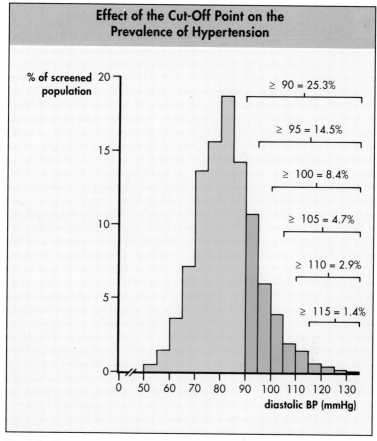

Fig. 3.2 Frequency distribution of diastolic blood pressures. Note the substantial increase in proportion of population defined as being hypertensive as the criterion for hypertension is lowered towards the population mean. (Modified from HDFP Cooperative (1977) *Circ Res*; **40**: I-106–I-109.)

subjects is therefore quite arbitrary (Fig. 3.1). As a consequence, lowering the criterion for diagnosing hypertension has a progressively greater effect upon the proportion of patients defined as hypertensive; the closer we get to the population mean (Fig. 3.2). Thus, altering the criterion from 100mmHg to 90mmHg may not have great significance for the individual patient but has a major impact on overall numbers.

Life expectancy is progressively reduced with increasing blood pressure due to the risk of death from cardiovascular disease (Fig. 3.3). Furthermore, the risks of systolic and diastolic blood pressure are additive, so that for any given systolic pressure, life expectancy diminishes as diastolic pressure increases and vice versa (Fig. 3.4). Systolic blood pressure becomes progressively more important than diastolic blood pressure with advancing age and for the elderly taking diastolic blood pressure into account adds little to using systolic blood pressure as a predictor of life expectancy. Just as there is no discreet dividing line between hypertensives and normotensives, so there is no dividing line between those blood pressures which are harmful and those which are not. Lower than average blood pressures are associated with better than average life expectancy unless very low pressures are a consequence of disease (Fig. 3.5). Hypertension cannot, therefore, be defined by simply considering subjects at risk either of dying, or of developing cardiovascular disease, as a result of high blood pressure.

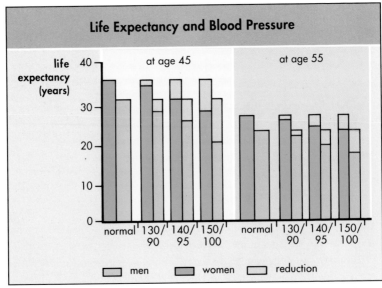

Fig. 3.3 Reduction in life expectancy produced by slight elevation of blood pressure.

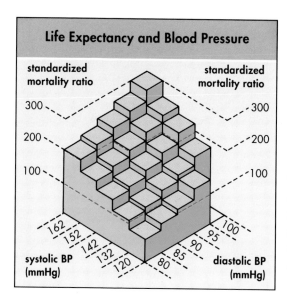

Fig. 3.4
Relationship between risk of death and blood pressure. Mortality risk is expressed as mortality ratio (population average = 100). (Modified from The Society of Actuaries (1959) *Build and Blood Pressure Study*, 1. Chicago: Society of Actuaries.)

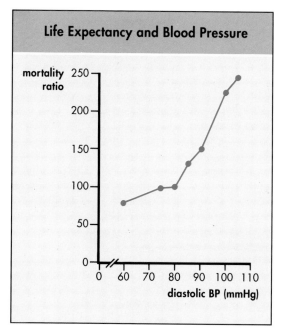

Fig. 3.5
Mortality ratio in relation to diastolic blood pressure in a healthy population. Lower diastolic blood pressures are associated with a better than average life expectancy. (Modified from The Society of Actuaries (1959) *Build and Blood Pressure Study*, 1. Chicago: Society of Actuaries.)

21

HYPERTENSIVE MORBIDITY

The risks associated with hypertension are due to vascular disease affecting the brain, heart, peripheral vessels and kidneys. The relative risks for specific organ disease vary according to patients' age and sex. Thus, hypertension (defined as a blood pressure of 160/95 mmHg or above) was associated with an increased risk, varying between 5 and 30 times, in different age and sex groups in the Framingham Study. Overall, in the Framingham Study, hypertensive patients were seven times as likely to develop a stroke (Fig. 3.6), six times as likely to develop congestive

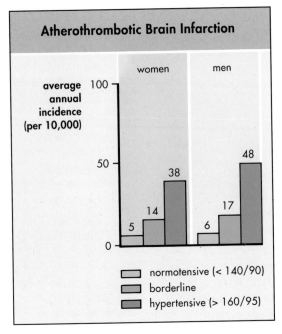

Fig. 3.6 Risk of stroke (atherothrombotic brain infarction) in the Framingham Study. (Modified from Kannel & Sorlie (1975) *Epidemiology and Control of Hypertension*. New York: Stratton.)

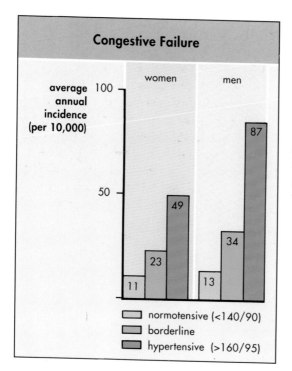

Fig. 3.7 Risk of congestive cardiac failure in the Framingham Study. (Modified from Kannel & Sorlie (1975) *Epidemiology and Control of Hypertension.* New York: Stratton.)

cardiac failure (Fig. 3.7), four times as likely to develop coronary heart disease (Fig. 3.8) and twice as likely to develop peripheral arterial disease (Fig. 3.9) as normotensive individuals.

The risk of dying as a result of hypertensive nephropathy is much smaller and largely confined to patients with the most severe forms of hypertension. With the advent of effective antihypertensive treatment, terminal renal disease directly due to hypertension has decreased, although poorly controlled hypertension contributes to accelerated decline of renal function in primary renal disease.

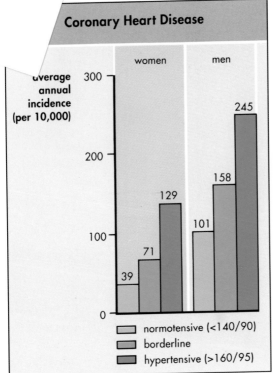

Fig. 3.8 Risk of coronary heart disease in the Framingham Study. (Modified from Kannel & Sorlie (1975) *Epidemiology and Control of Hypertension*. New York: Stratton.)

The risk of developing major cardiovascular disease increases by approximately 30% for each 10mmHg rise in systolic blood pressure in men and women of all ages. The lower relative risk for heart disease, as compared with stroke, is probably due to the greater importance of other risk factors (such as smoking and hypercholesterolaemia) in causing coronary heart disease. As a result of the weaker relationship for coronary heart disease, treatment of hypertension, even if risk were completely reversed, would not produce such a large proportionate fall in incidence of coronary heart disease compared with the predicted fall in stroke incidence. However, since coronary heart disease is much more common than stroke, the absolute benefit resulting from reversal of risk is greater for coronary heart disease than for stroke.

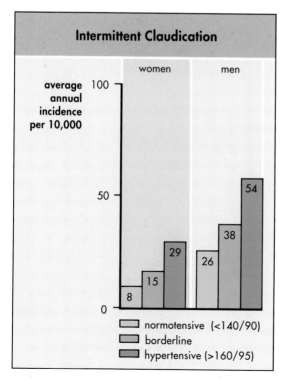

Fig. 3.9 Risk of intermittent claudication in the Framingham Study. (Modified from Kannel & Sorlie (1975) *Epidemiology and Control of Hypertension.* New York: Stratton.)

EFFECT OF TREATMENT ON RISK

There has been a dramatic improvement in prognosis of accelerated (malignant) hypertension with treatment. Whilst more than 90% of patients had died within a year, before effective antihypertensive medication became available, the five year survival rate for accelerated hypertension is now over 80%. Early studies, such as that conducted by the Veterans Administration, confirmed the unequivocal benefits of treating moderate and severe hypertension (diastolic blood pressure of 115 mmHg and above), although benefits were largely confined to reduction in cerebrovascular accident, congestive cardiac failure and renal damage (Fig. 3.10).

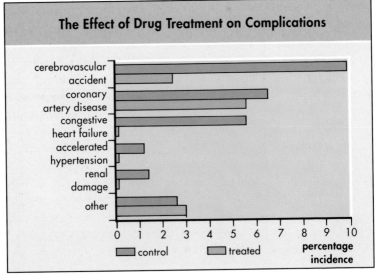

Fig. 3.10 Effect of drug treatment on the incidence of complications in moderate to severe hypertension – the Veterans Study. (Modified from Veterans Study (1970) *J Am Med Assoc*; **213**: 1143–1152.)

Blood Pressure Reduction		
	stroke	CHD
predicted decrease (observational studies)	35–40%	20–25%
observed decrease (clinical trals)	42±6%	14±5%

Fig. 3.11 Comparison of predicted decrease in strokes and coronary heart disease (from observational studies) and observed decrease in clinical trials of treatment in mild hypertension. Note complete reversibility of hypertension related stroke risk. (Modified from McMahon et al. (1990) Lancet; **335**: 768.)

The impact upon coronary heart disease was much less. A number of trials have examined the benefits in patients with mild hypertension (diastolic blood pressure of 90–100mmHg). Meta-analysis of these trials has shown that the average fall in diastolic blood pressure of 6mmHg would produce a reduction in incidence of stroke of 35–40%, if the risk attributable to hypertension was totally reversed. The observed reduction averaged 42%, indicating that the risk of stroke, attributable to hypertension, could in fact be totally eliminated. The impact on coronary heart disease was less evident, i.e. an observed reduction of 14% compared with a predicted reduction of 24% (Fig. 3.11).

The reason for this shortfall is unknown. The most likely explanation is that any benefits in terms of ischaemic heart disease are only observed after longer periods of treatment than those employed in the clinical trials. It has also been suggested that adverse metabolic effects of diuretics or β-blockers might have increased susceptibility to ischaemic heart disease. There are no direct comparative trials to clarify this, although reported changes in cholesterol and potassium are too small to support this explanation.

Most of the large trials have recruited patients on the basis of diastolic blood pressure. Systolic blood pressure is, however, a more important risk factor in the elderly. The Systolic Hypertension in the Elderly Programme

(SHEP) trial recruited patients with a systolic blood pressure of 160mmHg or more and a diastolic blood pressure of 90mmHg or more. Treatment (diuretic first line, atenolol second line) produced significant impact, both upon stroke (decreased by 36%) and coronary heart disease (decreased by 27%) (Fig. 3.12). It appears, therefore, that the risk associated with systolic hypertension is as readily reversible as that associated with diastolic hypertension.

CLINICAL ASSESSMENT

The mercury manometer is still the standard method for blood pressure measurement. Aneroid manometers require regular standardization. The sitting blood pressure is adequate for routine measurement, although

SHEP Trial			
	Active treatment	Placebo	Reduction
Coronary heart disease	140	184	27%
Stroke	199	289	36%
Cardiovascular disease	289	414	32%

Systolic hypertension in the elderly (SHEP) trial in isolated systolic hypertension showed a significant reduction in stroke and coronary heart disease.

Fig. 3.12   The Systolic Hypertension in the Elderly Programme (SHEP) trial in isolated systolic hypertension shows a significant reduction in stroke and coronary heart disease.

lying and standing blood pressures are necessary when postural hypotension is being sought. Blood pressure should, on the first occasion, be measured in each arm using a cuff which extends along at least two-thirds of the circumference of the upper arm. The cuff should be approximately at the level of the heart and pressure raised at least 10mmHg above that at which the radial pulse disappears on palpation. Pressure should be released steadily at a rate of 5mmHg per second and the point of disappearance of Korotkoff sounds (Phase V) taken as the measure of diastolic pressure. In patients with a high output state, the sounds may persist to zero and Phase IV Korotkoff (muffling) has then to be used for diastolic blood pressure (Figs 3.13 & 3.14). Phase IV measurements are usually 5–10mmHg higher than Phase V.

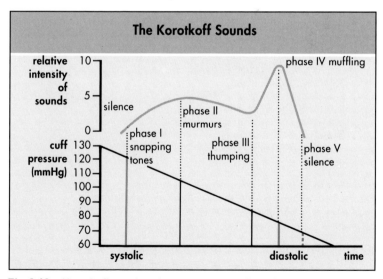

Fig. 3.13 Korotkoff sounds in the measurement of blood pressure.
Appearance of sounds provides a good measure of systolic blood pressure whilst diastolic blood pressure may be taken either as the point of sudden muffling of sounds (Phase IV) or at their disappearance (Phase V).

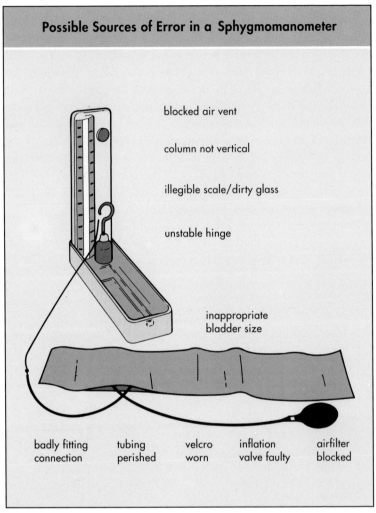

Fig. 3.14 Possible sources of error using a sphygmomanometer.

Ambulatory (24-hour) blood pressure monitoring has not yet reached routine clinical use. It is, however, valuable in diagnosing patients who have a pressor response to blood pressure measurement (white coat hypertension) (Fig. 3.15). If 24-hour blood pressure monitoring is not available, where this is suspected, patients should be loaned an electronic sphygmomanometer for home blood pressure measurement.

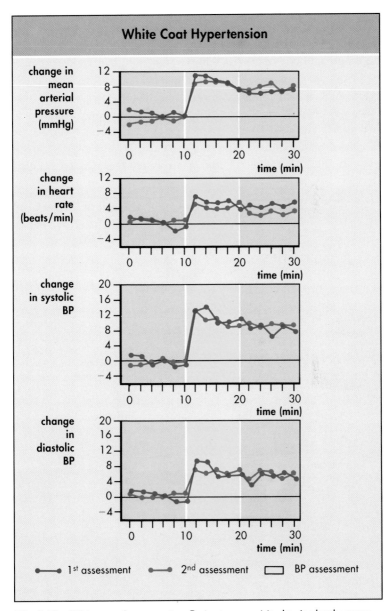

Fig. 3.15 White coat hypertension. Patients were visited twice by the same doctor. Each visit had the same marked effect raising both systolic and diastolic blood pressures, with a small increase in heart rate. (Modified from Mancia *et al.* (1983) *Lancet*; **ii**: 695–698.)

Clinical history taking and examination is directed at finding evidence of target organ damage or a possible primary cause of hypertension (Fig. 3.16). It should be emphasized, however, that in most cases hypertension is an asymptomatic condition. It is particularly important to detect evidence of ischaemic heart disease, cardiac failure, peripheral vascular disease and hypertensive retinopathy (Fig. 3.17). Secondary hypertension is unusual. The most common cause, i.e. the contraceptive pill, can be diagnosed on the basis of history. Coarctation is suspected on clinical grounds (Fig. 3.18). Other forms of secondary hypertension, such as

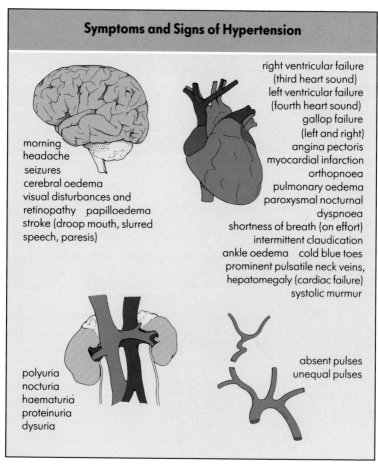

Symptoms and Signs of Hypertension

morning headache
seizures
cerebral oedema
visual disturbances and retinopathy   papilloedema
stroke (droop mouth, slurred speech, paresis)

right ventricular failure (third heart sound)
left ventricular failure (fourth heart sound)
gallop failure (left and right)
angina pectoris
myocardial infarction
orthopnoea
pulmonary oedema
paroxysmal nocturnal dyspnoea
shortness of breath (on effort)
intermittent claudication
ankle oedema   cold blue toes
prominent pulsatile neck veins, hepatomegaly (cardiac failure)
systolic murmur

polyuria
nocturia
haematuria
proteinuria
dysuria

absent pulses
unequal pulses

Fig. 3.16 Symptoms and signs suggesting target organ damage in hypertension.

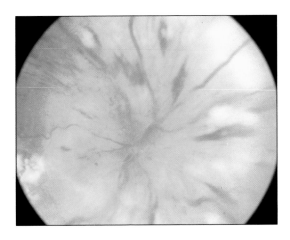

Fig. 3.17 Gross papilloedema, flame haemorrhages, cotton wool exudates and retinal oedema in a patient with malignant hypertension.

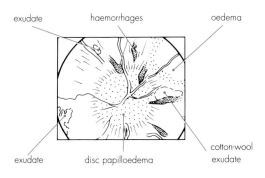

exudate   haemorrhages   oedema

exudate   disc papilloedema   cotton-wool exudate

Fig. 3.18 Major symptoms and signs in coarctation of the aorta.

Signs and Symptoms of Coarctation

systolic murmur over back and collaterals	arterial neck pulsation
large left ventricle	radial/femoral delay
rib notches (on x-ray)	cold feet
claudication	

Renal Disorders Associated with Hypertension

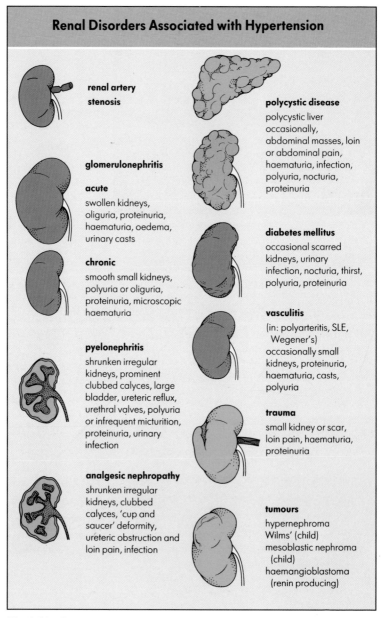

renal artery
stenosis

glomerulonephritis

acute

swollen kidneys,
oliguria, proteinuria,
haematuria, oedema,
urinary casts

chronic

smooth small kidneys,
polyuria or oliguria,
proteinuria, microscopic
haematuria

pyelonephritis

shrunken irregular
kidneys, prominent
clubbed calyces, large
bladder, ureteric reflux,
urethral valves, polyuria
or infrequent micturition,
proteinuria, urinary
infection

analgesic nephropathy

shrunken irregular
kidneys, clubbed
calyces, 'cup and
saucer' deformity,
ureteric obstruction and
loin pain, infection

polycystic disease

polycystic liver
occasionally,
abdominal masses, loin
or abdominal pain,
haematuria, infection,
polyuria, nocturia,
proteinuria

diabetes mellitus

occasional scarred
kidneys, urinary
infection, nocturia, thirst,
polyuria, proteinuria

vasculitis

(in: polyarteritis, SLE,
Wegener's)
occasionally small
kidneys, proteinuria,
haematuria, casts,
polyuria

trauma

small kidney or scar,
loin pain, haematuria,
proteinuria

tumours

hypernephroma
Wilms' (child)
mesoblastic nephroma
 (child)
haemangioblastoma
 (renin producing)

Fig. 3.19 Renal disorders associated with hypertension. Renal disease is responsible for high blood pressure in a minority of cases. Here, symptoms, signs and nephrological appearances which may suggest the diagnosis are shown.

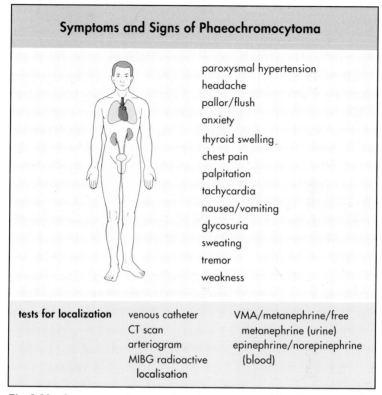

Symptoms and Signs of Phaeochromocytoma

paroxysmal hypertension
headache
pallor/flush
anxiety
thyroid swelling
chest pain
palpitation
tachycardia
nausea/vomiting
glycosuria
sweating
tremor
weakness

tests for localization	venous catheter	VMA/metanephrine/free
	CT scan	metanephrine (urine)
	arteriogram	epinephrine/norepinephrine
	MIBG radioactive	(blood)
	localisation	

Fig. 3.20 Symptoms and signs of phaeochromocytoma. Not all are present but the most common are headache, pallor, sweating, palpitations and nausea. Flushing occurs after the initial pallor. Possible sites for the tumour, apart from the adrenal gland, range from the pelvis to the upper thorax.

renovascular disease and renal disease (Fig. 3.19), phaeochromocytoma (Fig. 3.20) and primary aldosteronism (Fig. 3.21) should only be intensively sought if a clinical clue is present in the form of symptoms, unusual age of onset or abnormalities on routine screening of renal function or electrolytes (Fig. 3.22).

Clinical Features of Primary Aldosteronism

muscle weakness

cramps and tetany

polyuria

low serum K^+

high normal or high serum Na^+

high serum HCO_3^-

Fig. 3.21 Clinical clues which may suggest primary aldosteronism. Compare with secondary aldosteronism (due to diuretics or severe hypertension) where potassium is low, bicarbonate elevated, but serum sodium low or low/normal.

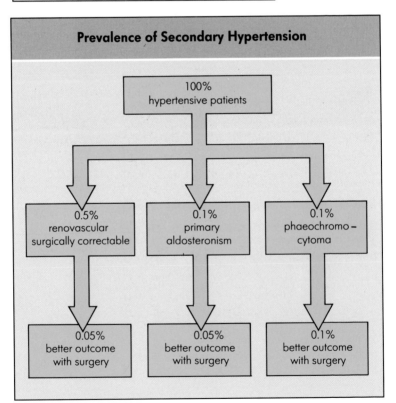

Prevalence of Secondary Hypertension

100%
hypertensive patients

0.5%
renovascular
surgically correctable

0.1%
primary
aldosteronism

0.1%
phaeochromo–
cytoma

0.05%
better outcome
with surgery

0.05%
better outcome
with surgery

0.1%
better outcome
with surgery

Fig. 3.22 In unselected populations screening for major forms of secondary hypertension changes management in very few patients. Intensive search for a cause, therefore, should be confined to those in whom there is a clinical suspicion.

MANAGEMENT

Immediate treatment is indicated only in the presence of serious complications, i.e. haemorrhages, exudates or papilloedema on fundal examination or left ventricular failure, hypertensive encephalopathy or dissecting aneurysm (Fig. 3.23). In other cases, blood pressure should be measured on two or three occasions before treatment is begun since in most cases a fall in blood pressure will be observed with habituation to blood pressure measurement. The major problem in management of mild hypertension is the very large population of patients who are eligible for treatment. Two strategies have to be adopted:

- Low cost, low risk therapy, i.e. non-pharmacological treatment.
- Identification of high risk patients who stand to gain most from antihypertensive medication.

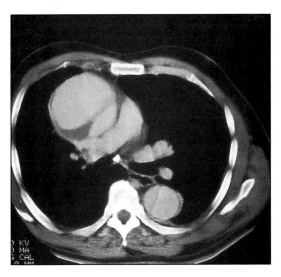

Fig. 3.23 CT scan of dissecting aneurysm of the aorta, showing dissection of the media by extravasated blood.

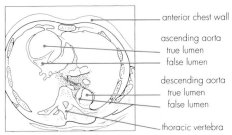

anterior chest wall

ascending aorta
true lumen
false lumen

descending aorta
true lumen
false lumen

thoracic vertebra

37

NON-PHARMACOLOGICAL THERAPY

This consists of:

- Body weight reduction in obese subjects. A 3 kg weight loss will produce a fall in blood pressure of 7/4 mmHg in a hypertensive patient (Fig. 3.24).
- Restriction of alcohol in heavy drinkers, i.e. in those who imbibe 6 or more units of alcohol per day, lowers blood pressure by about 1 mmHg for each unit of alcohol reduced (Fig. 3.25).

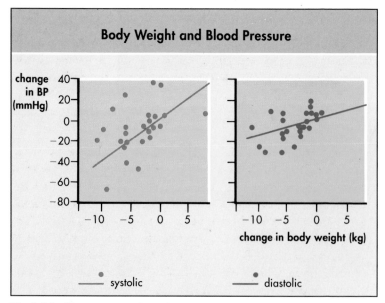

Fig. 3.24 Changes in systolic and diastolic blood pressure produced by changes in body weight in untreated hypertensive patients over one year. (Modified from Ramsey et al. (1978) *Br Med J*; 2: 244–245.)

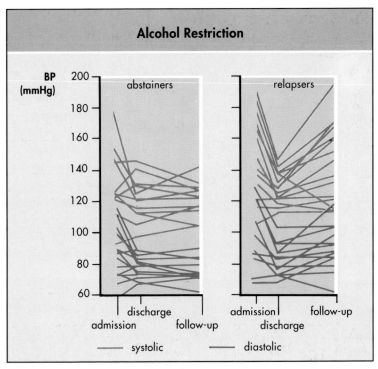

Fig. 3.25 Effects of alcohol restriction on systolic blood pressure and diastolic blood pressure in heavy drinkers following abstention and consequent relapse. (Courtesy of Dr G Beevers.)

- Moderate salt restriction from an average intake of about 150 mmol per day to 70–80 mmol per day reduces blood pressure in a subset of hypertensive patients (Fig. 3.26). It is particularly useful in patients receiving diuretic, β-blocker or converting enzyme inhibitor treatment. In untreated mild hypertension diastolic blood pressure falls of 1–4 mmHg can be expected on average, although individual variability is great. A greater response is seen with more severe hypertension.

- Physical training has a substantial blood pressure lowering effect. Regular daily training on a bicycle ergometer in one study produced a blood pressure fall greater than would be expected with β-blocker treatment (Fig. 3.27). Lesser degrees of exercise have a less pronounced effect on blood pressure.

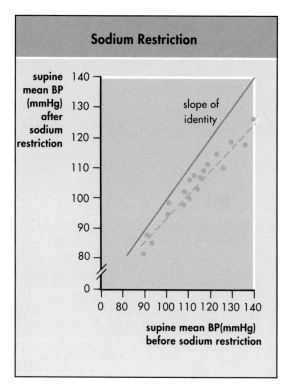

Fig. 3.26 Effect of moderate salt restriction on blood pressure in clinical trials of normotensive and hypertensive patients. Note that the largest blood pressure falls were observed in trials amongst more severely hypertensive patients.

- Biofeedback and relaxation exercises produce small falls in blood pressure (Fig. 3.28) but are extremely labour intensive and best reserved for patients who are enthusiastic about them.

Non-pharmacological therapy should be used in all patients who present with mild hypertension. In addition, all patients should be advised to stop smoking. Although this will have no effect upon blood pressure it is an extremely important additional risk factor.

IDENTIFICATION OF HIGH RISK PATIENTS

Drug treatment should be reserved for high risk hypertensive patients. The British Hypertension Society Working Party identified five criteria for such patients. These were as follows:

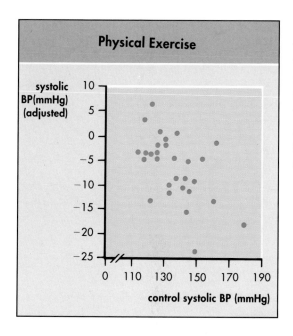

Fig. 3.27 Effect of regular physical exercise on blood pressure. Subjects undertook three training sessions per week over a period of one to eight months.

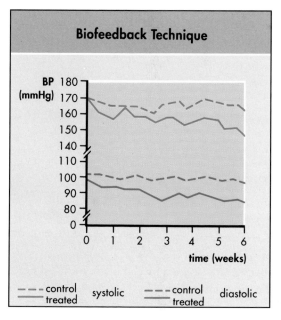

Fig. 3.28 Effect of biofeedback training on blood pressure in mildly hypertensive patients.

Blood Pressure Level

The greatest risk and therefore the greatest rewards for treatment are observed in patients with diastolic blood pressure of 100mmHg or more. In the MRC study of patients with a diastolic blood pressure of 90–109mmHg, for instance, more than three times as many strokes were prevented in patients with a diastolic blood pressure of 100mmHg or more compared with those whose initial blood pressure was below 100mmHg (see Fig. 3.3).

Repeated Measurement of Blood Pressure over a Prolonged Period

Average diastolic blood pressures of 100mmHg or more in the Australian Therapeutic Trial were associated with much higher incidence of trial end points such as stroke or myocardial infarction (Fig. 3.29). Regular blood pressure measurement over at least a three month period is

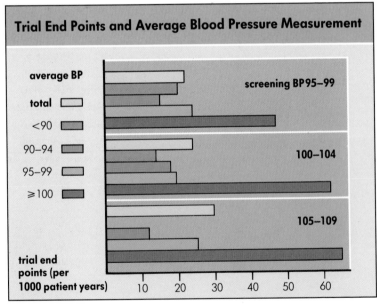

Fig. 3.29 Average blood pressure was a much better predictor of outcome during the three years of the Australian Therapeutic Trial, compared with initial blood pressure (screening columns). Note that patients whose average diastolic blood pressure was 100mmHg or more were at much higher risk. Data from placebo group.

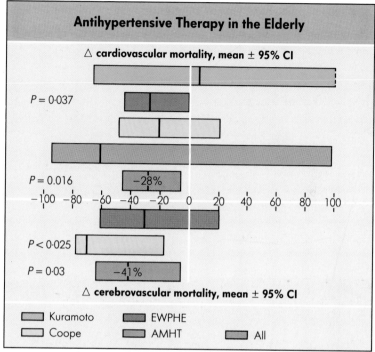

Fig. 3.30 Meta-analysis of trials of antihypertensive therapy in elderly people. The overall reduction in stroke mortality (41%) is very similar to that observed in younger patients. There is also, however, a reduction in cardiovascular mortality (28%) which is less marked in younger subjects. More recent trials; MRC, Hypertension in the Elderly and STOP–Hypertension, show similar results. (Modified from Staessen *et al. Eur Heart J* 1988; **9**: 215–222.)

therefore recommended in mild hypertension, although shorter periods are more appropriate for patients with presenting diastolic blood pressures above 110mmHg. If average diastolic blood pressure is 100mmHg or more, drug treatment should normally be used.

Age

The proportionate benefits of reducing blood pressure are retained in the elderly and since the absolute risk of cardiovascular disease is much higher, the individual benefits are correspondingly higher, at least up to the age of 80 (Fig. 3.30). It should also be remembered, however, that the

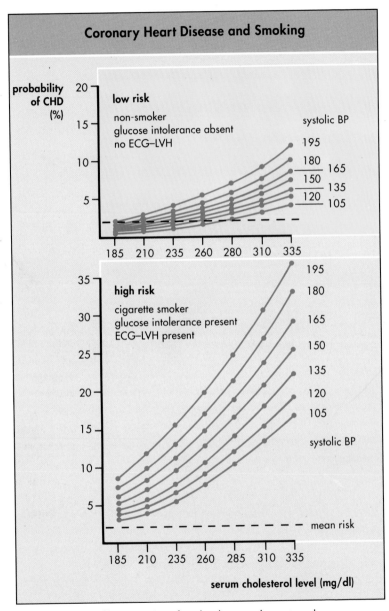

Fig. 3.31 Risks of hypertension of any level are much greater when concurrent risk factors are present. (Modified from Kannel & Kreger (1981) *Blood Pressure Measurement and Systemic Hypertension.* Edited by Arntzenius *et al.* Medical World Publishing.)

adverse effects of drugs are much more frequent in the elderly a
poorer compliance. Blood pressure reduction, therefore, has to be mor
gradual and blood pressure monitored more frequently.

Gender

The incidence of strokes and heart attacks is less in women than in
men, so that the absolute benefits of treatment are correspondingly less,
although the proportionate benefits are the same in both sexes.

Other Risk Factors

The multiplicative effects of other risk factors; left ventricular hypertrophy, glucose intolerance, hyperlipidaemia, and continued cigarette
smoking have been discussed (Fig. 3.31). Threshold for treatment should,
therefore, be lowered in these patients to 90 or 95mmHg (Fig. 3.32).

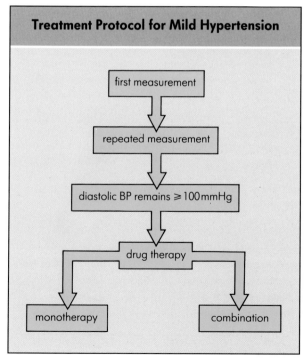

Fig. 3.32 Outline protocol for treating patients with mild hypertension on presentation, i.e. diastolic blood pressure 90–110mmHg.

TARGET TREATMENT

There is little to be gained by attempting to reduce diastolic blood pressure below 80–85 mmHg. There is some evidence that, in patients with pre-existing ischaemic heart disease, reducing blood pressure below these levels may actually be harmful (Fig. 3.33). The SHEP trial indicates

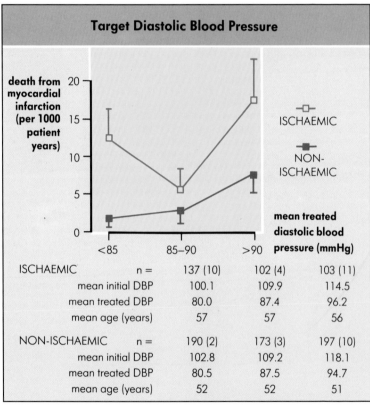

		<85	85–90	>90
ISCHAEMIC	n =	137 (10)	102 (4)	103 (11)
	mean initial DBP	100.1	109.9	114.5
	mean treated DBP	80.0	87.4	96.2
	mean age (years)	57	57	56
NON-ISCHAEMIC	n =	190 (2)	173 (3)	197 (10)
	mean initial DBP	102.8	109.2	118.1
	mean treated DBP	80.5	87.5	94.7
	mean age (years)	52	52	51

Fig. 3.33 In some studies, based upon surveys of hypertension clinics, patients with pre-existing heart disease have a higher mortality rate when diastolic blood pressure is reduced below 80–85 mmHg. The same phenomenon is also observed in untreated patients with ischaemic heart disease. How far treatment to lower blood pressure levels has a harmful effect is still debatable. (Modified from Cruickshank *et al. Lancet* 1987; 581–583.)

that systolic hypertension, even when unaccompanied by diastolic hypertension, should also be treated with a target reduction of systolic blood pressure to values below 160mmHg.

DRUG TREATMENT

All major classes of antihypertensive therapy are licensed as first line treatment. Selection of the most appropriate drug should be tailored to the particular patient (Fig. 3.34). Thus, β-blockers should normally be first line treatment in patients who suffer from angina or have previously sustained a myocardial infarct, whilst diuretics and ACE inhibitors are preferred agents in those who have a history of heart failure in association with hypertension. Afro-Caribbean blacks respond poorly to β-blockers and ACE inhibitor treatment. In other cases, there will be pharmacological contraindications, e.g. to β-blockers in patients with obstructive airways disease or diuretics in patients with gout. Under these circumstances first line treatment with an ACE inhibitor or α-adrenoceptor antagonist may be necessary.

Where there are no specific indications for a particular class of drug, choice will be dictated by individual patient tolerance and economic cost. Where monotherapy fails to control blood pressure, a second or even a third class of agent may be added as combination therapy. In this case, some classes of drugs are complementary and therefore provide the best combination (Fig. 3.35).

Options for Hypertension Drug Therapy

	Advantages	Disadvantages	Contra indications
Diuretics	Cheap Proven benefit in end-point trials Reduction of osteoporotic fractures	Adverse effects on lipids Insulin resistance Hypokalaemia Hyperuricaemia Impotence	Gout Non-insulin diabetes mellitus
β-Blockers	Proven benefit in secondary infarction Treatment of angina Proven benefit in end-point trials	Adverse effect on lipids Impotence Reduced effort tolerance Raynaud's phenomenon Ineffective in blacks Negative inotropic effect	Obstructive Airways disease Cardiac failure
α-Blockers	Beneficial effect on lipids	Hypotension Impotence	
ACE inhibitors	Improved outcome in cardiac failure	Cough Renal failure in impaired renal blood flow (e.g. bilateral renal artery stenosis) Hypotension in sodium depleted patients Ineffective in blacks	Bilateral renal artery stenosis or single kidney with renal artery stenosis
Dihydro-pyridine Ca channel blockers	Treatment of angina	Oedema Sympathetic NS stimulation	
Other Ca channel blockers e.g. verapamil diltiazem	Treatment of angina	Negative inotropic effect Constipation (verapamil)	Conduction disturbances

Fig. 3.34 Advantages and disadvantages of major classes of drug used in treating hypertension.

Options for Combination Therapy	
β-blocker:	calcium antagonist
β-blocker:	diuretic
ACE inhibitor:	diuretic
α-blocker:	β-blocker/ calcium antagonist
ACE inhibitor:	calcium antagonist

Fig. 3.35 Popular combinations in treating hypertension. These are used when monotherapy fails.

Lipids

BIOCHEMISTRY

Lipids are a heterogenous class of chemicals characterized by insolubility in water and solubility in organic solvents such as chloroform or ether. They have two major functions.

- Energy storage and transport. They are particularly efficient as their calorie value is twice that of carbohydrates.
- Structural. They are the major components of membranes, which separate aqueous compartments within and between cells and prevent the free diffusion, therefore, of water-soluble solutes.

LIPID CLASSES

There are three classes of lipids: triglycerides, phospholipids and cholesterol.

Triglycerides

Three long-chain fatty acids are attached to a glycerol skeleton.

Phospholipids

These have a similar structure to triglycerides but, instead of the fatty acid in position 3, there is a phosphate-containing molecule such as phosphatidylcholine or phosphatidylethanolamine. This constitutes the polar head of the molecule which is charged and hydrophilic. The non-polar fatty acid end of the molecule is hydrophobic. Different physical properties of the two ends render phospholipids an essential structural component of cell membranes and lipid protein complexes.

Cholesterol

Cholesterol is a steroid molecule, which is polar in the free state, but in plasma about 75% of the cholesterol is esterified.

LIPOPROTEINS

Lipids are transported in spherical complexes with apolipoproteins (apo-proteins) (Fig. 4.1). These proteins contain helical regions which are hydrophobic at one end and hydrophilic (charged) at the other. The charged polar head groups of the phospholipids and alcohol groups of unesterified cholesterol project from the surface of the lipoprotein particle into the plasma. The non-polar part of the phospholipid and apolipo-protein molecule lie in the core of the particle which also contains esterified cholesterol and triglyceride.

The density of the lipoprotein complex depends upon its protein component. They are separable by ultracentrifugation into five groups, performing different biochemical functions (Fig. 4.2).

LIPID TRANSPORT

There are two pathways of lipid transport.

EXOGENOUS PATHWAY

Cholesterol and fatty acids derived from dietary fat are re-esterified into triglycerides and synthesized into chylomicrons. These are metabolized to chylomicron remnants containing esterified cholesterol and the apo-proteins apo B-48 and apo E. The apo E is recognized by specific hepatic parenchymal receptors and removed from the bloodstream (Fig. 4.3).

ENDOGENOUS TRANSPORT

Fatty acids which are not oxidized by the liver are esterified to form triglycerides, but instead of being synthesized into chylomicrons, they are synthesized into VLDL with additional phospholipid and protein components. The VLDL is subsequently metabolized and VLDL rem-nants taken up by liver receptors or VLDL is metabolized to LDL which is then removed by specific hepatic LDL receptors. Extra-hepatic tissues remove smaller proportions of LDL (Fig. 4.4).

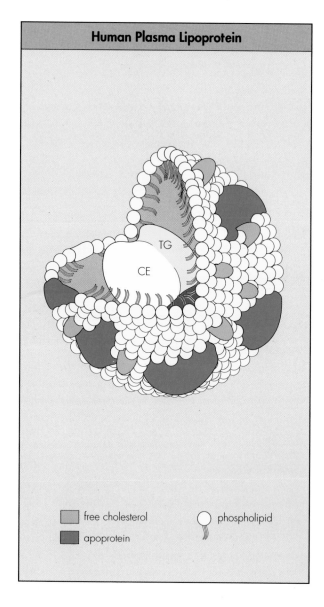

Human Plasma Lipoprotein

TG

CE

free cholesterol   ◯ phospholipid

apoprotein

Fig. 4.1
Structure of a plasma lipoprotein. Note that the hydrophobic lipid region of the molecule contains the free cholesterol and triglycerides, whilst the polar end of phospholipids and proteins lies on the outside.

The Density Classes of Plasma Lipoproteins				
	density (d; g/ml)	sources	electrophoretic mobility	mean diameter (nm)
chylomicrons CYHLO	<0.95	intestine	origin	500
very low VLDL density lipoproteins	<1.006	liver	pre-β	43
intermediate IDL density lipoproteins	1.006–1.019	catabolism of VLDL & chylomicrons	'broad β'	27
low density LDL lipoprotein	1.019–1.063	catabolism of VLDL	β	22
high density HDL lipoproteins	1.063–1.21	catabolism of chylomicrons & VLDL; liver & intestine	α	8

Fig. 4.2   Five major classes of lipoproteins which can be separated by ultracentrifugation.

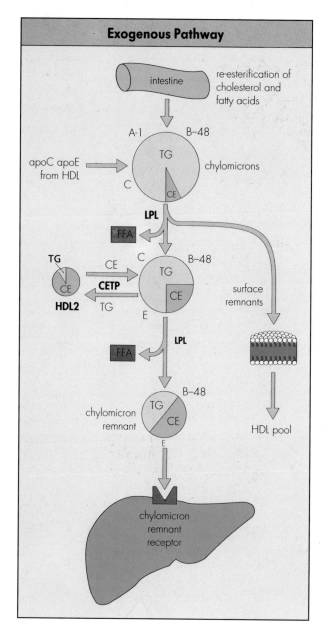

Fig. 4.3 The exogenous pathway of lipid transport.

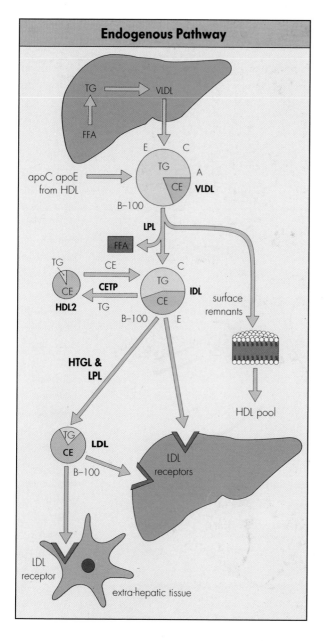

Fig. 4.4
The endogenous pathway of lipid transport.

LIPIDS AS RISK FACTORS

The clinical importance of lipids as risk factors is their association with atheroma. The atheromatous plaque incorporates lipoprotein taken up into the arterial wall (Fig. 4.5).

CHOLESTEROL

Both within and between populations there is a highly significant association between total plasma cholesterol and coronary heart disease (Fig. 4.6). There is strong evidence in favour of a causal relationship. Thus,

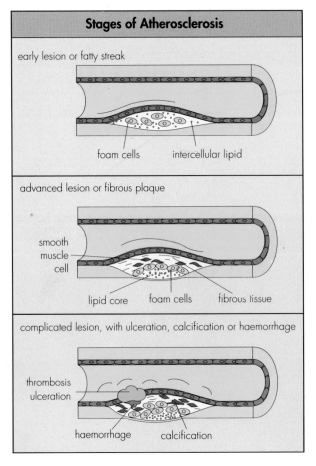

Stages of Atherosclerosis

early lesion or fatty streak

foam cells   intercellular lipid

advanced lesion or fibrous plaque

smooth muscle cell

lipid core   foam cells   fibrous tissue

complicated lesion, with ulceration, calcification or haemorrhage

thrombosis ulceration

haemorrhage   calcification

Fig. 4.5 Evolution of the atheromatous plaque. Note, that, at an early stage, lipid containing foam cells are present although the final episode in vascular occlusion is probably haemorrhage through a fissure in the plaque.

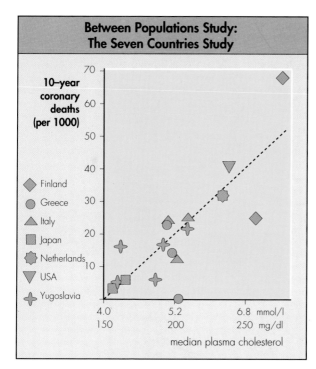

Between Populations Study: The Seven Countries Study

10–year coronary deaths (per 1000)

◆ Finland
● Greece
▲ Italy
■ Japan
⬡ Netherlands
▼ USA
✛ Yugoslavia

4.0 / 150   5.2 / 200   6.8 mmol/l / 250 mg/dl

median plasma cholesterol

Fig. 4.6 Between populations study: the Seven Countries study. In this study involving 12,763 men in 16 different regions from seven countries, the median cholesterol levels were highly correlated with CHD mortality. (Modified from Keys A, Seven Countries. Harvard University Press, 1980.)

Migration Study			
	Japan	**Hawaii**	**San Francisco**
cholesterol mmol/l	4.7	5.6	5.9
mg/dl	181	218	228
CHD rate per 1000	25.4	34.7	44.6

Fig. 4.7 Migration study; cholesterol levels and CHD rates in Japanese living in Japan, Hawaii and San Francisco. (Modified from Nichamen MZ et al. Am J Epidemiol 1975; **102**: 2823–2828.)

when changes in diet, associated with migration, cause plasma cholesterol to rise the incidence of coronary heart disease also rises (Fig. 4.7). Reduction in high cholesterol levels by diet and drugs also gives rise to a reduction in coronary heart disease.

The relationship between plasma cholesterol and coronary heart disease is a continuous one. The majority of subjects whose plasma cholesterol lies close to the population mean, therefore, are at increased risk compared with individuals who have the lowest cholesterol (Fig. 4.8).

Assuming that the cholesterol associated risk is reversible at these levels, as well as at the highest plasma cholesterol levels, there are very substantial benefits obtainable from a population reduction in cholesterol levels, provided that the methods used do not themselves increase morbidity.

CHOLESTEROL SUBFRACTIONS IN CORONARY HEART DISEASE

LDL-cholesterol is more closely associated with coronary heart disease than total cholesterol. This is consistent with the view that uptake of LDL (or oxidized LDL) is an important pathogenetic process (Fig. 4.9). Conversely, HDL-cholesterol is inversely associated with the risk of coronary heart disease, i.e. low HDL-cholesterol is associated with increased risk and vice versa.

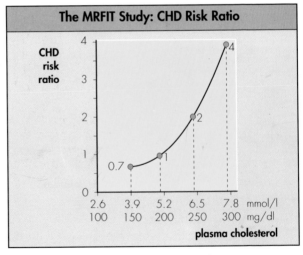

Fig. 4.8 Lowest CHD rates occur when cholesterol is 5.2mmol/l (200mg/dl) or below. The risk of CHD is doubled at 6.5mmol/l (250mg/dl) and quadrupled at 7.8mmol/l (300mg/dl). (Modified from Martin MJ et al. Lancet 1986; ii: 933–936, and Stamler J, Wentworth D, Neaton J JAMA 1986; 256: 2823–2828.)

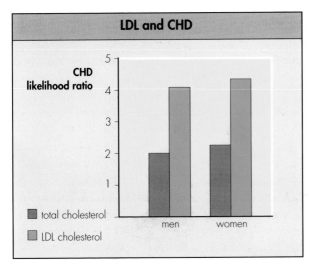

Fig. 4.9 Likelihood ratios for CHD with respect to total cholesterol and LDL-cholesterol in the Framingham Heart Study.

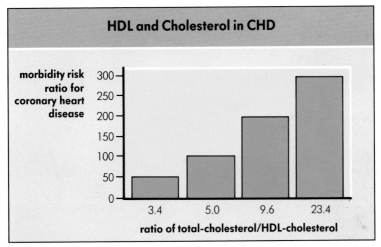

Fig. 4.10 The Framingham Study: Four-year risk of coronary heart disease according to the ratio of cholesterol lipoprotein fractions. (Modified from Kannel WB *Nutrition Rev* 1988; **46**: 68.)

Since the risks associated with these different cholesterol fractions are independent, better assessment of risk is provided by the ratio of LDL-cholesterol/HDL-cholesterol or total cholesterol/HDL-cholesterol. A ratio, in the latter case, of 4.5 is associated with the population average risk of coronary heart disease, i.e. a risk ratio of 1 (Fig. 4.10).

APOLIPOPROTEINS

LDL contains mainly apo B and HDL contains mainly apo A (Fig. 4.11). High levels of apo B and low levels of apo A have been shown in some studies to be associated with higher incidence of coronary heart disease than the respective lipoproteins. However, the predictive value of these apoproteins has not been established by longitudinal follow-up studies.

LIPOPROTEIN A

This is an LDL-like particle which is elevated in some subjects with coronary heart disease. It is structurally similar to plasminogen and its importance may possibly lie, therefore, in a putative role in the thrombotic cascade.

TRIGLYCERIDES

Triglycerides are a positive risk factor for coronary heart disease (Fig. 4.12). However, they are associated with other risk factors such as total cholesterol, LDL-cholesterol, body mass index and blood pressure. How far they are an independent risk factor, when these other factors are taken into account, is controversial. However, in clinical practice, they are useful in identifying high risk patients. Severe hypertriglyceridaemia

Apoproteins and CHD	
apoA and apoB	in cross-sectional studies apoA-I and apoB have been shown to be better discriminators for the presence of coronary disease than their respective lipoproteins HDL and LDL the predictive value of these apoproteins for subsequent CHD has not been established
Lp(a)	Lp(a), an LDL-like particle, containing apoB-100 and apo(a), is elevated in subjects with CHD apo(a) is structurally similar to plasminogen, indicating that this particle has a potential role in thrombogenesis as well as atherogenesis

Fig. 4.11 Other biochemical risk factors related to plasma lipids.

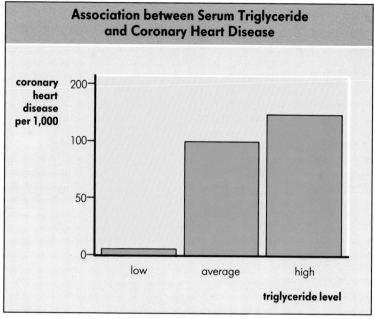

Fig. 4.12 The Framingham Study: The association between the levels of serum triglyceride and incidence of coronary heart disease in men with low levels of HDL-cholesterol < 1.0mM (40mg/dl); low triglyceride < 1.1mM (94mg/dl); average triglyceride 1.1–1.6mM (94–114mg/dl); high triglyceride > 1.6mM (> 145mg/dl). (Modified from Castelli WP *Am Heart J* 1986; **112**: 432.)

(more than 6.0mmol/l or 500mg/dl) may give rise to a hypercoagulable state, whilst very high serum triglycerides (more than 11.0mmol/l or 1000mg/dl) may cause pancreatitis.

THE HYPERLIPIDAEMIAS

PRIMARY HYPERLIPIDAEMIA

The primary hyperlipidaemias are essentially genetic disorders, although diet may modify their phenotypic expression (Fig. 4.13). In non-specialist clinical practice, the most likely causes are familial hypercholesterolaemia, familial combined hyperlipidaemia and polygenic hypercholesterolaemia (Figs 4.14 & 4.15).

Phenotyping of Hyperlipoproteinaemias

phenotype	lipoprotein abnormality	major plasma lipid elevation	minor plasma lipid elevation
I	chylomicrons	triglycerides	cholesterol
IIa	LDL (β)	cholesterol	
IIb	LDL (β) and VLDL (pre-β)	cholesterol and triglycerides	
III	IDL (β)	cholesterol and triglycerides	
IV	VLDL (pre-β)	triglycerides	cholesterol
V	VLDL (pre-β) and chylomicrons	triglycerides	cholesterol

Fig. 4.13 Classification of hyperlipidaemias according to Fredrickson. Since this classification was put forward there has been much further information on the basis of lipid disorders. However, it still provides a useful classification based upon biochemical findings.

Primary Hyperlipidaemias

defect	site	disorder	lipoprotein abnormality	major lipid elevation
enzyme	lipoprotein lipase	lipoprotein lipase deficiency	chylomicrons	triglyceride
receptor	B, E receptor	familial hypercholesterolaemia	LDL	cholesterol
apoprotein	apoE	apoE-2 homozygosity (remnant hyperlipidaemia)	IDL	cholesterol, triglyceride
	apoC-II	ApoC-II deficiency	chylomicrons	triglyceride
defect uncertain		hyperalphalipo-proteinaemia	HDL	cholesterol
		familial hypertriglyceridaemia	VLDL (rarely chylomicrons)	triglyceride
		familial combined hyperlipidaemia	LDL, VLDL	cholesterol triglyceride
		polygenic hypercholesterolaemia	LDL	cholesterol

Fig. 4.14 Classification of hyperlipidaemias based upon knowledge (where it has been acquired) of the basic disorder.

Primary Hyperlipidaemias: Prevalence and Clinical Features

disorder	prevalence	transmission	clinical signs	clinical features	
				pancreatitis risk	atherosclerosis risk
lipoprotein lipase deficiency	very rare	autosomal recessive	hepatosplenomegaly, eruptive xanthomas, lipaemia retinalis	+	–
familial hypercholesterolaemia		autosomal dominant	corneal arcus, xanthelasmas, tendonous xanthomas		
homozygote	1:1,000,000		tuberous xanthomas	–	+++
heterozygote	1:500			–	++
apoE2 homozygosity	1:10,000	polygenic	palmar crease xanthomas, tuberous xanthomas, tubero-eruptive xanthoma	–	++
apoC-II deficiency	very rare	autosomal recessive	hepatosplenomegaly, eruptive xanthomas, lipaemia retinalis	+	–
hyperalphalipo-proteinaemia	varies	polygenic		–	–
familial hypertriglyceridaemia	1:600	autosomal dominant	in severe forms: hepatosplenomegaly, eruptive xanthomas, lipaemia retinalis	+	?+
familial combined hyperlipidaemia	1:300	?polygenic ?autosomal dominant	corneal arcus, xanthelasmas	–	++
polygenic hypercholesterolaemia	common	polygenic	corneal arcus, xanthelasmas	–	+

Fig. 4.15 Prevalence and clinical features of the primary hyperlipidaemias. Of the most common primary hyperlipidaemias, familial combined hyperlipidaemia, polygenic hypercholesterolaemia and familial hypertriglyceridaemia are seen in adulthood and often occur in the absence of clinical signs. In familial combined hyperlipidaemia the lipoprotein phenotype varies within families.

Familial hypercholesterolaemia (Fredrickson Type IIa)

This is due to impaired hepatic LDL receptors inhibiting the uptake of LDL and preventing the normal inhibition of cholesterol synthesis, produced by LDL, after it is taken up by the liver (Fig. 4.16). LDL receptor activity is absent in the homozygous condition, in which coronary heart disease occurs frequently during the second decade of life, whilst in the heterozygous condition, 50% of LDL receptors are present and coronary heart disease is delayed until the fourth or fifth decade.

Familial Hypercholesterolaemia		
	homozygote	**heterozygote**
cholesterol	usually > 15.5mmol/l 600mg/dl	usually > 7.8mmol/l 300mg/dl
clinical features:		
cutaneous	tendon xanthoma tuberous xanthomas	tendon xanthoma xanthelasma
corneal arcus	corneal arcus may be seen before 20 years	common
polyarthritis	during adolescence	uncommon
premature atherosclerosis	CHD often within 2nd decade aortic ejection murmur (from aortic root atheroma)	CHD within 4th–5th decade

Fig. 4.16 Characteristics of familial hypercholesterolaemia.

Familial combined hyperlipidaemia

This may have a variety of lipoprotein patterns, but in which cholesterol and triglyceride are both elevated, and is also associated with myocardial infarction and can be demonstrated in up to 30% of the families of patients with myocardial infarction. The genetic basis of the disorder and its pathogenesis have not been elucidated.

Causes of Secondary Hyperlipidaemia			
	lipid changes		
	cholesterol	triglyceride	HDL
conditions			
obesity	→↑	↑	↓
diabetes mellitus			
untreated	→↑	↑	↓
IDDM (treated)			→↑
NIDDM (treated)		↑	↓
hypothyroidism	↑		
chronic renal failure	→↑	↑	↓
nephrotic syndrome	↑	↑	↓
biliary obstruction	↑		
myeloma	↑	↑	
glycogen storage disease	↑		
drugs			
alcohol excess		↑	
thiazides	↑	↑	→↓
β-blockers		↑	↓
corticosteroids		↑	
oestrogens		↑	↑
progestagens	↑	↑	↓

Fig. 4.17 Causes of secondary hyperlipidaemia.

Polygenic hypercholesterolaemia

Usually Type IV or Type IIB, this is probably the commonest cause of elevated cholesterol in middle-aged and elderly subjects, reflecting interaction between several genes and environmental influences.

In considering genetic causes of hyperlipidaemia it is important to distinguish between rare genes of large effect, such as the gene for familial hypercholesterolaemia, and common genes of small effect, such as the genes which code for the different phenotypes of apo E. The population incidence of the familial hypercholesterolaemia gene is about 1 in 500, so although this gene has a marked effect on the health of its carriers, it contributes less than 1% to the total population burden of ischaemic heart disease.

Conversely, although an unfavourable apo E phenotype has only a small effect on the life expectancy of an individual, because these genes occur in up to 25% of the population, the effect on population morbidity and mortality is substantial.

SECONDARY HYPERLIPIDAEMIA

An adverse lipid profile is frequently observed as a consequence of either drug therapy or other medical conditions (Fig. 4.17). In some of these conditions there is a well demonstrated increased risk of coronary heart disease, e.g. diabetes, chronic renal failure and nephrotic syndrome. In other situations, e.g. myeloma, the duration of the illness may not be sufficient for the patient to exhibit increased risk.

ASSESSMENT OF HYPERLIPIDAEMIC PATIENTS

Patients may present either as a result of screening or because of development of target organ damage (Fig. 4.18). Assessment involves a full clinical history, specifically enquiring about target organ damage, full family history and with a complete examination (Figs 4.19–4.24). Where familial hyperlipidaemia is suspected, first degree relatives should also have lipids measured.

Fasting specimens are essential for measurements of triglycerides, but total or HDL-cholesterol can be measured on non-fasting specimens (Fig. 4.25). Where one of the rarer causes of primary hyperlipidaemia is suspected, measurements of the relevant apoprotein or lipoprotein lipase activity or LDL receptor activity can be undertaken in specialist laboratories.

Recommendations for Individual Assessment

history

personal history of hyperlipidaemia or CHD
  age of onset?
  treatment?

family history of hyperlipidaemia, CHD or peripheral vascular disease
  in first-degree relative (parent or sibling)
  or second-degree relative
  age of onset?

known hypertension, diabetes mellitus, hypothyroidism?
alcohol consumption?
tobacco: number of cigarettes smoked? duration?
other medication?
current diet?

examination

weight
weight and height for body mass index (BMI) calculation
$$BMI = weight\ (kg) \div [height\ (m)]^2$$
blood pressure

corneal arcus, xanthelasmas, xanthomas (cutaneous, palmar, tendons)?

pulses
features of hypothyroidism, diabetes, etc.

laboratory investigation

fasting lipids: total cholesterol, TG and HDL

glucose
liver function test
γGT
creatinine   to exclude/confirm
urinary protein   secondary
thyroid function tests   hyperlipidaemia
haemoglobin blood count and film

Fig. 4.18 Recommendations for individual assessment.

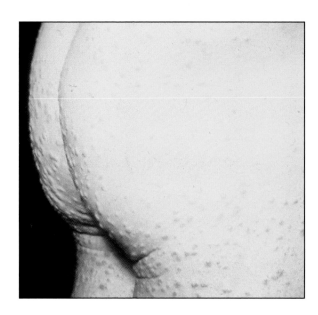

Fig. 4.19
Eruptive
xanthomas
are a feature
of the familial
chylomicron-
aemia
syndrome.
(Courtesy of
Dr RS
Elkeles,
London.)

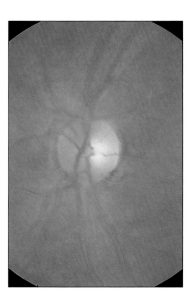

Fig. 4.20
Lipaemia retinalis in
a patient with
familial hyper-
triglyceridaemia,
Fredrickson Type I.
Note the milky-
white appearance
of the retinal blood
vessels due to
dilution with fat-
containing particles.
(Courtesy of Dr D
Galton, St
Bartholomew's
Hospital, London.)

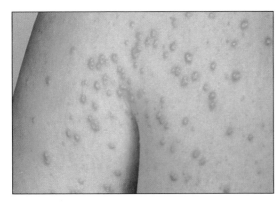

Fig. 4.21 Crops of eruptive xanthomata appearing over the skin of a patient with familial hyperlipidaemia. (Courtesy of Dr D Galton, St Bartholomew's Hospital, London.)

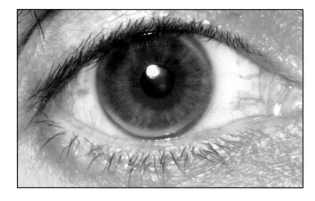

Fig. 4.22 Corneal arcus commonly occurs in hypercholesterolaemia, as well as in older people. (Courtesy of Dr MD Feher, Charing Cross and Westminster Medical School, London.)

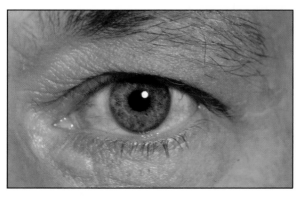

Fig. 4.23 Eyelid xanthelasma are commonly seen in normocholesterolaemic subjects. (Courtesy of Dr MD Feher, Charing Cross and Westminster Medical School, London.)

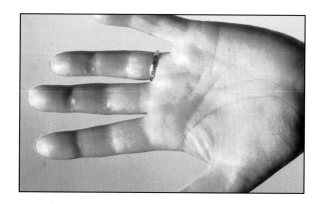

Fig. 4.24 Palmar crease xanthomas. (Courtesy of Dr RS Elkeles, London.)

Recommendations: The Patient

12-h fast preferred but not essential for total or HDL cholesterol

Patient should be seated for at least 5 minutes

Avoid stasis (if needed a tourniquet should be applied for the minimum of time)

Maintain habitual diet including alcohol – weight should be stable

---

defer: 2 weeks after minor illness
2–3 months after myocardial infarction
2–3 months after illness or pregnancy

---

a sample drawn within 24h of onset of myocardial infarction may match the pre-infarction state

two measurements c. 1 month apart are required to reliably assess cholesterol status

serial measurements should be performed using the same laboratory

Fig. 4.25   Recommendations for laboratory measurements: the patient.

TREATMENT OF HYPERLIPIDAEMIA

EFFECT OF CHOLESTEROL LOWERING

It cannot be assumed that the risk associated with disturbances in plasma lipids can be corrected by reversal of lipid abnormality. Endpoint trials are extremely difficult and costly since relatively large populations of subjects have to be followed for prolonged periods of time. Trials have inevitably focussed on high risk subjects where benefits are likely to be greatest. Available evidence, therefore, relates only to patients with elevated cholesterol levels. These have shown benefit in the form of a reduction of coronary heart disease (Fig. 4.26a) and in the rate of progression of atheroma, assessed angiographically (Fig. 4.26b).

Studies have not shown a reduction in total mortality. It should be borne in mind, however, that they were not designed for this purpose and much larger trials would be needed to show an impact upon overall death rates, since death from other causes will dilute an effect upon cardiovascular mortality. It has been suggested that the failure to show an impact upon death rate is due to lipid lowering therapy actually increasing death from other causes. In the absence of adequate trial data this remains speculative.

GUIDELINES

Lipid disorders are managed by dietary control and in selected cases drug treatment. The decision to treat is based upon assessment of the individual patient's risk, determined by measurement of plasma lipids and the presence of target organ damage and other risk factors.

It is important to treat the whole patient and not just the hyperlipidaemia. As pointed out in other chapters, hyperlipidaemia interacts strongly with other risk factors, such as hypertension and smoking. Persuading a hyperlipidaemic patient to stop smoking may improve his survival prospects more than correcting the hyperlipidaemia.

SERUM LIPIDS AND TREATMENT

Since the relationship between risk and plasma cholesterol is continuous, there is no biological threshold at which treatment is indicated. The threshold for treatment is the level at which potential benefits are outweighed by the risk and cost of treatment, both in terms of money and inconvenience. In general, the lower the plasma cholesterol the lower

Lipid Modification in Relation to CHD	number in study	duration (years)	treatment	lipid response (%) ↓ chol	↓ TG	↑ HDL	reduction in CHD incidence (%)
primary prevention trials							
LA Veterans study	846	8	diet alone	13			23
WHO Cooperative Trial of Clofibrate	15,745	5	clofibrate	9			20
Lipid Research Clinics Coronary Primary Prevention Trial (LRC-CPPT)	3806	7.4	cholestyramine	13			19
Helsinki Heart Study	4081	5	gemfibrozil	11	35	34	34
secondary prevention trials							
Coronary Drug Project (niacin group)	3908	5	niacin	10			26
Stockholm Ischaemic Heart Disease Secondary Prevention Study	555	5	clofibrate + nicotinic acid	13	19		36

Fig. 4.26a Effect of lipid modification upon clinical coronary artery disease and angiographic assessment of atheromatous plaques. Note that the primary prevention trials studied patients with hyperlipidaemia, whilst the secondary prevention trials and the angiographic trials studied patients with established atheroma. There have been no primary prevention trials in patients with lipid levels which are only modestly elevated.

Lipid Modification with Angiographic Assessment

	number in study	duration (years)	treatment	lipid response (%) ↓ chol	↓ TG	↑ HDL	angiographic outcome (progression/regression)
coronary artery disease							
Finnish Regression Study	28	7	clofibrate + nicotinic acid	18	38	10	↓ progression
NHLBI Type II Coronary Intervention Study	116	5	cholestyramine	15		8	↓ progression
Cholesterol-Lowering Atherosclerosis Study (CLAS)	162	2	colestipol + niacin	26		37	↓ progression 16% regression
Familial Atherosclerosis Study (FATS)	103	2.5	colestipol + lovastatin	LDL ↓ 48		14	↓ progression >10% regression
			colestipol + nicotinic acid	LDL ↓ 34		41	↓ progression >10% regression
femoral artery disease							
Duffield et al.	24	1.7	cholestyramine nicotinic acid, or clofibrate	25	45	25	60% ↓ progression

Fig. 4.26b Effect of lipid modification upon clinical coronary artery disease and angiographic assessment of atheromatous plaques.

the risk, although the marginal benefits of reduction in plasma cholesterol become very small in subjects at the lower end of the population range.

Some epidemiological studies have shown a slight excess of mortality, due to deaths from malignant disease, in the bottom quintile of plasma cholesterol. Whether this is due to a causal relationship between low cholesterol and predisposition to malignancy or whether, as seems more likely, early malignancy has an effect upon plasma cholesterol, is still debatable. Since the plasma cholesterol concentrations at which this phenomenon has been demonstrated are well below the target levels for treatment, these observations have no practical bearing on treatment of hypercholesterolaemia.

Specialist bodies in Europe (Fig. 4.27) and the USA (Figs 4.28 & 4.29) have issued guidelines on the treatment of hyperlipidaemia. Although there are important differences between guidelines issued by different bodies, the underlying principle is the same, i.e. the use of diet for managing patients at mildly increased risk and the use of drugs and diet for patients whose risk is more substantial. The USA guidelines recommend further analysis of lipoprotein subclass in patients with elevated cholesterol. This, it is suggested, avoids unnecessary treatment of patients with high cholesterol but a low LDL/HDL ratio.

DIET

Overweight patients should restrict total calorie intake until they have attained their 'ideal' bodyweight. Calorie restriction will reduce plasma triglycerides in all patients and cholesterol in polygenic/obesity related hyperlipidaemia (Fig. 4.30). It will also improve diabetic control in obese maturity onset diabetics. Slim patients with hypercholesterolaemia invariably have a genetic rather than an environmental cause for it. Reduction in the proportion of energy derived from fats (to less than 30%) and in the proportion of saturated to unsaturated fats will also reduce plasma cholesterol. Although diets very high in polyunsaturated fats have sometimes been recommended, there is a worry that because unsaturated fatty acids are susceptible to peroxidation in the vessel wall, they may actually promote the development of atheroma.

Dietary advice should also include advice on increasing the intake of fresh fruit and vegetables, as these are valuable sources of biological antioxidants, such as vitamin C and carotene. Individuals vary widely in the extent to which plasma cholesterol reflects dietary cholesterol intake,

Management of Hypercholesterolaemia: European and UK Guidelines

cholesterol		assessment	management
mmol/l	mg/dl		
5.2–6.5	200–250	assess overall risk of CHD taking into account risk factors and younger age	correct overweight correct other modifiable risk factors advise dietary improvement
6.5–7.8	250–300	assess overall risk of CHD, taking into account risk factors and younger age	correct overweight correct other modifiable risk factors prescribe lipid-lowering diet drug treatment, if response inadequate and other risk factors present
>7.8	>300	assess overall risk of CHD, taking into account risk factors and younger age and consider referral to specialist clinic	correct overweight correct other modifiable risk factors prescribe lipid-lowering diet likely to require drug treatment

Fig. 4.27 Summary of European and UK guidelines for management of hypercholesterolaemia. Intervention guidelines are based on total cholesterol levels and risk factor assessment.

Management of Hypercholesterolaemia: USA Guidelines			
initial assessment		**management and follow-up**	

	total cholesterol mmol/l (mg/dl)	management and follow-up	
without CHD and without 2 other risk factors	<5.2 (<200)	repeat total cholesterol within 5 years	
	5.2–6.2 (200–239)	dietary information and recheck annually	
with CHD or with 2 other CHD risk factors	5.2–6.2 (200–239)	lipoprotein analysis; then take further action based on LDL cholesterol levels	
	≥6.2 (≥240)		

assessment	LDL cholesterol mmol/l (mg/dl)	suggested treatment	minimum of therapy: LDL cholesterol mmol/l (mg/dl)
without CHD and without 2 other risk factors	≥4.1 (≥160)	diet	<4.1 (<160)
	≥4.9 (≥190)	diet + drug	<4.1 (<160)
with CHD or with 2 other CHD risk factors	≥3.4 (≥130)	diet	<3.4 (<130)
	≥4.1 (≥160)	diet + drug	<3.4 (<130)

Fig. 4.28 Summary of USA guidelines for management of hypercholesterolaemia. The guidelines are based on total cholesterol to assess risk, and on LDL-cholesterol to determine treatment and set therapeutic goals.

Management of Hypercholesterolaemia with Hypertriglyceridaemia

cholesterol triglyceride mmol/l (mg/dl)		assessment	management
5.2–7.8 (200–300)	2.3–5.6 (200–500)	assess overall risk of CHD, taking into account risk factors and younger age seek cause of raised lipids	correct overweight correct underlying cause and risk factors prescribe lipid-lowering diet drug treatment, if response inadequate and other risk factors present
>7.8 (>300)	>5.6 (>500)	assess overall risk of CHD, taking into account risk factors and younger age seek cause of raised lipids consider referral to specialist clinic	likely to require drug treatment correct overweight correct underlying cause and risk factors prescribe lipid-lowering diet

Fig. 4.29 Recommendations for management of hypercholesterolaemia with hypertriglyceridaemia; elevation of both serum cholesterol and triglyceride (combined hyperlipidaemia) is a common disorder. UK, European and USA guidelines are similar.

Lipid-Lowering Diet: General Advice

1. Attain ideal body weight; reduce energy intake, or increase energy expenditure by exercise
2. Reduce total fat to ≤30% of total dietary energy intake
3. Fat reduction: reduce saturated (mainly animal) fat to <10% of total energy
   partially replace saturated fat by monounsaturated and polyunsaturated fats (vegetable, olive and fish oils)
4. Reduce dietary cholesterol to <300mg/day
5. Increase intake of complex carbohydrates and soluble fibres (fruit, cereals, vegetables)

Fig. 4.30   Lipid-lowering diet: general advice.

but restricting cholesterol intake is sensible. Advice on weight loss, increased exercise and a healthy diet is appropriate for all hyperlipidaemic patients.

Drug therapy should be reserved for those with severe familial hyperlipidaemia, a poor family history, or as part of secondary prevention in patients with known ischaemic heart disease.

DRUGS

The different classes of lipid lowering drugs act at different sites in lipid metabolism (Fig. 4.31). In addition, some, such as the bile acid sequestrants, probucol and statin derivatives have an action upon cholesterol, whilst others such as fish oil, have an action solely upon plasma triglycerides (Fig. 4.32). The fibrates and nicotinates have an action on both lipids.

Selection of agents is, therefore, based upon the type of lipidaemia, patient tolerance of medication and efficacy (Figs 4.33 & 4.34). The bile acid resins require patients to take up to nine sachets per day, whilst vasodilator side effects of the nicotinates may limit dosage. Patients may, therefore, find compliance more difficult with these agents than with other cholesterol lowering drugs. Where single drug therapy is insufficient, combinations may have to be used (Figs 4.35 & 4.36). The

Mechanism of Action of Lipid-Regulating Therapy

	mechanism of action
diet	
reduce: cholesterol saturated fats	promotes receptor-mediated uptake of LDL
calorie reduction	decreases synthesis of VLDL
drug	
bile acid sequestrants	block bile acid reabsorption activate cholesterol oxidation to bile acids promote receptor-mediated uptake of LDL
HMG CoA reductase inhibitors	inhibit action of HMG CoA reductase, leading to enhanced receptor-mediated uptake of LDL
fibric acid derivatives	activate LPL and inhibit HMG CoA reductase, to increase VLDL catabolism and receptor-mediated uptake of LDL
probucol	antioxidant effect on LDL promotes non-receptor-mediated uptake of LDL decreases synthesis of HDL
nicotinic acid and derivatives	inhibit fatty acid release from adipocytes inhibit VLDL synthesis and secretion
fish oils	inhibit VLDL synthesis and secretion

Fig. 4.31   Lipid-lowering drugs: mechanism of action.

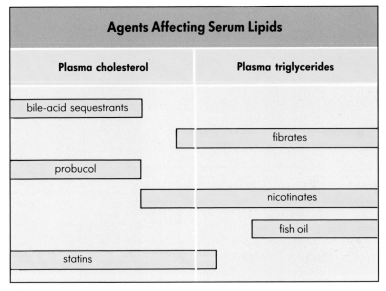

Fig. 4.32 Agents grouped according to whether their predominant action is on serum cholesterol or triglycerides.

Drug Groups used for Familial Lipid Disorders	
disorder	drug groups
hypercholesterolaemia	bile acid sequestrants fibric acid derivatives nicotinic acid derivatives probucol HMG CoA reductase inhibitors
combined hyperlipidaemia	fibric acid derivatives nicotinic acid derivatives HMG CoA reductase inhibitors
endogenous hypertriglyceridaemia	fibric acid derivatives nicotinic acid derivatives fish oils (pharmacological doses)
apoE-2 homozygosity	fibric acid derivatives nicotinic acid derivatives

Fig. 4.33 Drug groups used for familial lipid disorders.

81

Drug Therapy for Lipid Disorders

drug group + examples	dosage range	adverse effects	contraindications
bile acid sequestrants cholestyramine colestipol	2–6 × 4g 2–6 × 5g	abdominal discomfort, constipation, diarrhoea, may decrease absorption of other drugs, triglyceride elevation	elevated plasma triglycerides, complete biliary obstruction, peptic ulcer, pregnancy
fibric acid derivatives bezafibrate fenofibrate gemfibrozil	3 × 200mg or 1 × 400mg 3 × 100mg or 1 × 250mg 1–2 × 600mg	abdominal discomfort, nausea, rash, myalgia, may enhance effects of anticoagulants	severe liver or renal impairment, gallbladder disease, nephrotic syndrome, hypersensitivity, pregnancy
HMG CoA reductase inhibitors lovastatin* pravastatin simvastatin	20–80mg 10–40mg 10–40mg	flatulence, raised liver & muscle enzymes (± myopathy), rash	impairment of liver function, hypersensitivity, pregnancy, breast feeding
nicotinic acid and derivatives nicotinic acid (niacin) acipimox	1–3 × 1–2g 1–3 × 250mg	flushing, pruritus, nausea, glucose-intolerance (not observed with acipimox), dyspepsia, hyperuricaemia	impairment of liver function, congestive heart failure, recent myocardial infarction, gout, pregnancy, breast feeding, peptic ulcer, hypersensitivity
probucol	1–2 × 500mg	nausea, abdominal pain, prolonged QT interval, sweat odour, rash	impairment of liver function, biliary obstruction, pregnancy, breast feeding, arrhythmia
fish oils	1–10g	nausea, flatulence	peptic ulcer
*not currently in UK			

Fig. 4.34 Drug therapy for lipid disorders.

Monotherapy				
	lipids (% change)		lipoproteins (% change)	
	cholesterol	triglyceride	LDL	HDL
bile acid sequestrants	15–30	5–30	15–30	3–8
fibric acid derivatives	10–20	30–50	20–25	10–25
HMG CoA reductase inhibitors	20–33	10–30	25–45	2–15
nicotinic acid and derivatives	15–30	20–60	15–40	10–20
probucol	5–15	0–5	8–15	10–25
fish oils	↑ variable ↓	10–60	↑ variable	5–10
□ increase		□ decrease		□ variable

Fig. 4.35 Expected changes (%) in lipids and lipoproteins at optimal dosage of a single drug (monotherapy).

Drug Combinations	
drug combination	expected reduction in LDL-cholesterol (%)
bile acid sequestrant + nicotinic acid derivative	32–55
bile acid sequestrant + fibric acid derivative	25–40
bile acid sequestrant + probucol	25–40
bile acid sequestrant + HMG CoA reductase inhibitor	52–55
HMG CoA reductase inhibitor + nicotinic acid derivative	49–55
bile acid sequestrant + HMG CoA reductase inhibitor + nicotinic acid derivative	60–70

Fig. 4.36 Drug combinations. Cholesterol lowering can be greatly enhanced by using combinations of drugs that have different and complimentary mechanisms of action.

combination of fibrate and statins is not recommended as rhabdomyolysis is more frequent than with the individual drugs (Fig. 4.37).

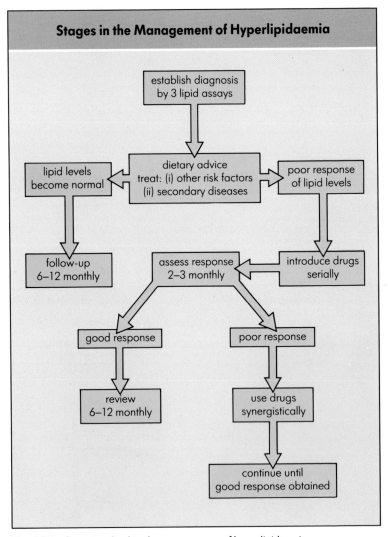

Fig. 4.37   Steps involved in the management of hyperlipidaemia.

OTHER MEASURES

Partial ileal bypass surgery is occasionally used for treating severe hyper-cholesterolaemia which cannot be controlled with drugs. The procedure interrupts the enterohepatic circulation of bile acids and results in the excretion of substantial amounts of cholesterol in the faeces, with a major fall in plasma cholesterol.

Plasma exchange (plasmapheresis) or selective binding of LDL-lipoproteins, in a haemoperfusion column, has been used extensively in homozygous familial hypercholesterolaemia where drug treatment is insufficient to lower plasma cholesterol to acceptable levels. Liver trans-plantation has also been carried out in patients with homozygous familial hypercholesterolaemia, to restore hepatic parenchymal LDL receptors.

PHYSICAL ACTIVITY

There is a relationship between the level of physical activity and coronary heart disease (Fig. 4.38). Thus, habitual exercise has been shown to be associated with a low risk of coronary heart disease amongst several groups of manual and white-collar workers in the USA and the UK.

Physical Activity and First Heart Attack			
	Physical activity in adult life*		
University athlete	Low	Medium	High
No	71	53	35
Yes	93	45	35
*levels of activity: low = <500 kcal/week; medium = 500–1999 kcal/week; high = >2000 kcal/week.			

Fig. 4.38 First heart attack rate (per 10,000 person-years) among male graduates from Harvard, during a six to ten year follow-up period. (Modified from Paffenberger RS *et al. Am J Epidemiol* 1978; **108**: 161–175.)

This appears to be independent of smoking, obesity, blood pressure or a family history of ischaemic heart disease. The mode of action of exercise is still uncertain. Apart from weight and blood pressure reduction, exercise results in an increase in HDL-cholesterol, reduction in triglycerides and reduction in insulin resistance.

In addition, exercise has a euphoriant action, probably related to secretion of endogenous opioids. The level of exercise necessary to achieve optimal benefit is still controversial, but moderate, regular exercise is desirable as part of advice for healthy living, not merely in individuals at high risk of cardiovascular disease.

OBESITY

Overweight patients are at increased risk of both coronary artery disease and stroke (Fig. 4.39). As in the case of blood pressure and lipids, the relationship is a continuous one so that subjects with a bodyweight below the population average have a particularly low risk of cardiovascular disease. The relationship is not straightforward, however, since bodyweight is associated with blood pressure, serum lipids and physical activity. When the relationship between bodyweight and risk is adjusted for these other factors, the effect of obesity on cardiovascular risk is no longer present. In other words, obesity is acting through these factors.

Nevertheless, the importance of correction of obesity on cardiovascular risk cannot be overestimated. The effects upon blood pressure, lipids and insulin resistance are discussed elsewhere. Because weight is related to physique as well as obesity, bodyweight is an unsatisfactory measure of obesity. Either body mass index (height^2/weight) or preferably ideal weight (see Chapter 5) should be used to define target weight.

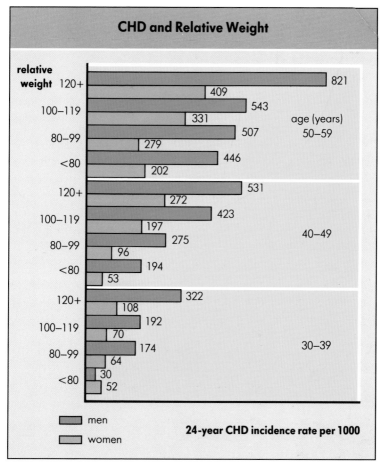

Fig. 4.39 Incidence of coronary heart disease according to relative weight (i.e. normal = 100). (Modified from Dawber TR. The Framingham Study; The Epidemiology of Atherosclerotic Disease. Cambridge, Harvard University Press, USA (1980).)

Diabetes and Glucose   5

DIABETES AS A CARDIOVASCULAR RISK FACTOR

Diabetic patients are at increased risk of atheroma, arterial calcification macrovascular complications (Fig. 5.1). In addition there is diabetic microvascular disease, with thickened capillary basement membranes and microaneurysm formation in small capillaries and venules (Fig. 5.2). Increased death rate from cardiac and renal disease accounts for the shortened life expectancy in diabetic patients (Figs 5.3–5.7).

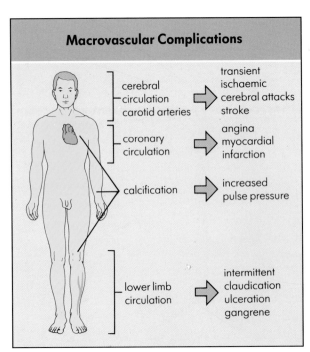

Macrovascular Complications

cerebral circulation carotid arteries → transient ischaemic cerebral attacks stroke

coronary circulation → angina myocardial infarction

calcification → increased pulse pressure

lower limb circulation → intermittent claudication ulceration gangrene

Fig. 5.1 Macrovascular complications in diabetes.

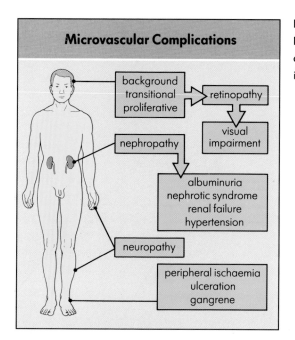

Fig. 5.2 Microvascular complications in diabetes.

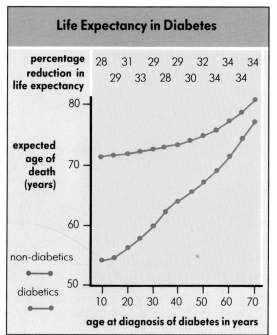

Fig. 5.3 Life expectancy is reduced by about one third in diabetics, at whatever age the disease is diagnosed. (Modified from Marks HH & Krall LP *Joslin's Diabetes Mellitus* Philadelphia (1971) Lea & Febiger.)

Diabetic Cardiovascular Death Rates		
Cause of death	**Death rate ratios for the diabetic to general population**	
	Males	**Females**
Total vascular disease	2.4	3.4
Aged 15–44 years	12.2	19.5
Aged 45–74 years	2.2	3.2
Heart disease	2.0	3.2
Cerebrovascular disease	1.8	2.0
Renovascular disease	17.8	17.0

Fig. 5.4 Death rates, relative to a healthy population, from specific cardiovascular causes in diabetics. These data were obtained from diabetics first diagnosed in the Joslin clinic between 1950 and 1958 and followed up to 1961. (Modified from Marks HH & Krall LP *Joslin's Diabetes Mellitus* Philadelphia (1971) Lea and Febiger.)

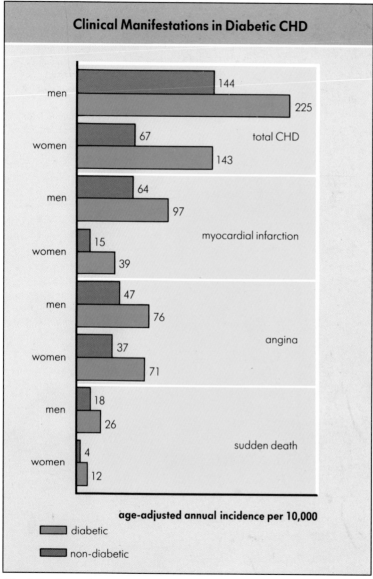

Fig. 5.5 Coronary heart disease and sudden death in diabetic and non-diabetic populations, followed up for 18 years in the Framingham Study. (Modified from Kannel WB *Diabetes and the Heart* Zonereich S (ed.) Thomas Springfield (1978).)

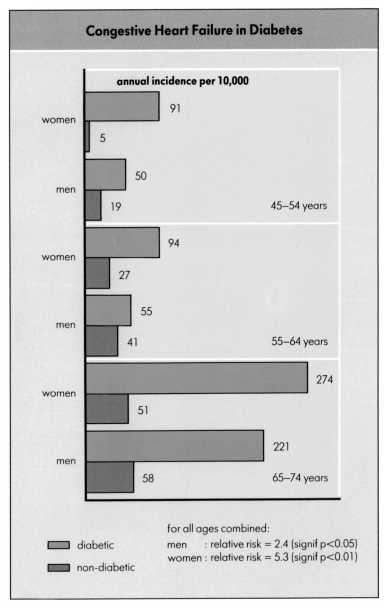

Fig. 5.6 Annual incidence of congestive heart failure in diabetic and non-diabetic men and women aged 45 to 74 years, followed up for 18 years in the Framingham Study. (Modified from Kannel WB *Diabetes and the Heart* Zonereich S (ed.) Thomas Springfield (1978).)

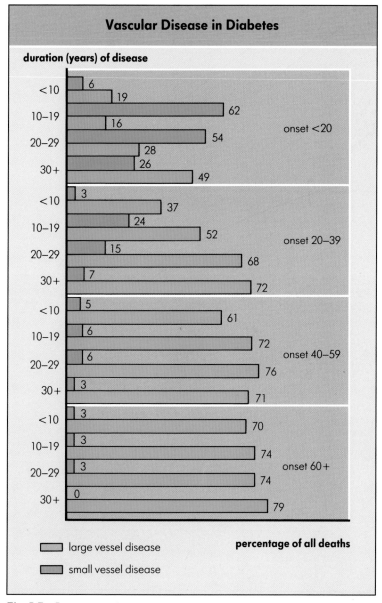

Fig. 5.7 Percentage of deaths due to microvascular and macrovascular disease in different age groups in the Joslin clinic. (Modified from Entmacher et al. *Diabetes* 1964;**13**:373.)

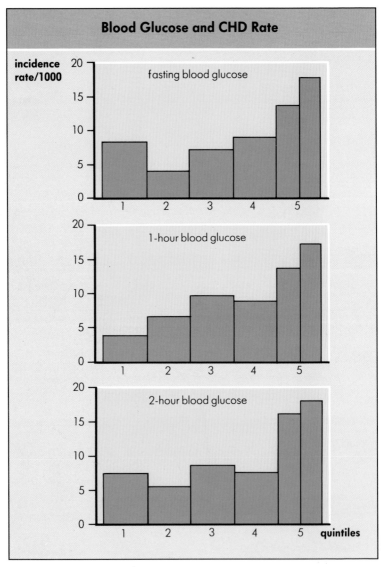

Fig. 5.8 Incidence of death from coronary heart disease or non-fatal myocardial infarction in 982 healthy men aged 35 to 64 years. Note that higher quintiles of fasting glucose or blood glucose, after a glucose load, were associated with a higher incidence of coronary heart disease in men. Data taken from the Helsinki Policemen Study. (Modified from Pyörälä K et al. INSERM Symp. 22 Amsterdam, Elsevier Biomedical Press (1982).)

There is also a relationship between glucose tolerance and coronary heart disease. Subjects whose blood glucose lies in the upper 20% of the population have increased risk of subsequent coronary heart disease (Fig. 5.8). The severity of cardiovascular disease also tends to be greater. Thus, mortality following myocardial infarction is greater in diabetics than in the general population (Fig. 5.9).

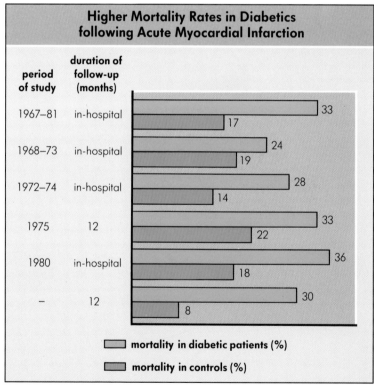

Fig. 5.9 Data from six independent studies showing higher mortality amongst diabetic patients following acute myocardial infarction. (Modified from Watson RDS and Waldron S *Diabetes and the Heart* Taylor KG (ed.) Castle House Publications, Tunbridge Wells (1987).)

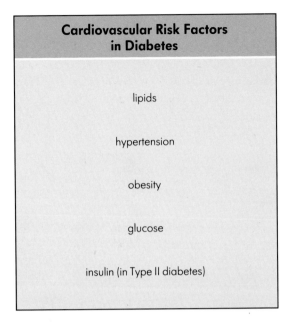

Fig. 5.10 Major risk factors associated with diabetes.

Cardiovascular Risk Factors in Diabetes

lipids

hypertension

obesity

glucose

insulin (in Type II diabetes)

Lipid Abnormalities

	Type I diabetes	Type II diabetes
Lipids	Hypertriglyceridaemia	Hypertriglyceridaemia
	Hypercholesterolaemia	Hypercholesterolaemia
Lipoproteins	Increased LDL	Increased LDL
	Increased VLDL	Increased VLDL
	Increased LDL-triglyceride	Increased LDL-triglyceride
	Normal or elevated HDL	Normal or reduced HDL

Fig. 5.11 Major abnormalities in circulating lipids found in untreated Type I and Type II diabetes.

RISK FACTORS IN DIABETES

There is a clustering of risk factors in diabetics and patients with impaired glucose tolerance (Fig. 5.10). Thus, Type II (non-insulin-dependent) diabetics are most likely to be obese, hypertensive and have an adverse serum lipid profile (Fig. 5.11). Conversely, hypertensive patients are more likely to have impaired glucose tolerance. This is independent of whether they have been treated with thiazide diuretics or not.

Both genetic and environmental factors contribute to this clustering of abnormalities (Fig. 5.12). Detailed family histories in Salt Lake City,

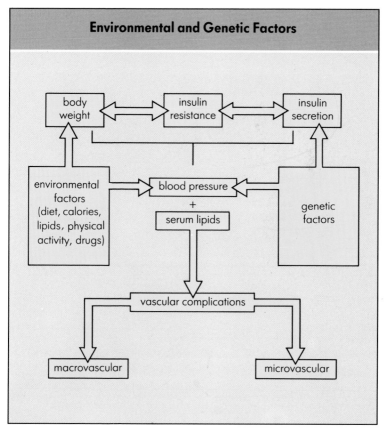

Fig. 5.12 Associations between major environmental and genetic risk factors in patients with insulin resistance.

Utah have identified the syndrome of familial combined hyperlipidaemia (dyslipidaemia) in which adverse serum lipid changes (increased LDL and triglycerides, together with decreased HDL-cholesterol) are associated with hypertension and insulin resistance (Fig. 5.13). It is suggested that high insulin levels (as a result of insulin resistance) cause elevated blood pressure, perhaps through increased sympathetic nervous system activity, sodium retention or perhaps acting as a trophic factor in resistance vessels.

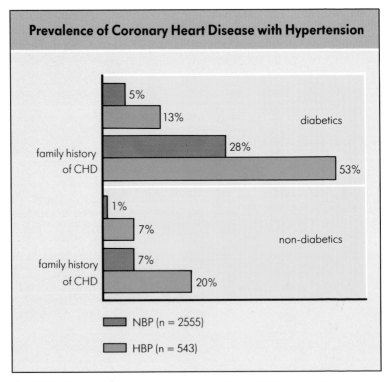

Fig. 5.13 Data from the Utah study obtained from 3098 subjects. Note that the presence of a family history of coronary heart disease and high blood pressure together, worsen prognosis amongst diabetics. Positive family history of coronary heart disease was significantly associated with dyslipidaemia. (Modified from Williams RR et al. Hypertension is an insulin-resistant disorder: genetic factors and cellular mechanisms. Elsevier Press; Amsterdam (1991): 89–101.)

Although there is undoubtedly a strong genetic component in the association of insulin resistance, hypertension and hyperlipidaemia, environmental factors are extremely important. When Australian Aborigines move to an urban environment they show a similar metabolic picture with obesity, insulin resistance, hyperlipidaemia and increased blood pressure. This is reversed when they revert to their traditional hunter–gatherer lifestyle (Fig. 5.14).

Environment and CHD Risk Factors in Aborigines

	Before	After 7 weeks	
Body weight (kg)	81.9±3.4	73.8 ± 2.8	$p<0.001$
Body mass index (kg/m)	27.2±1.1	24.5±0.8	$p<0.001$
Fasting glucose (mmol/l)	11.6±1.2	6.6±0.5	$p<0.001$
2-hr glucose	18.5±1.3	11.9±0.9	$p<0.001$
Fasting insulin (mU/l)	23±3	12±1	$p<0.005$
2-hr insulin	49±9	59±11	n.s.
Fasting triglycerides (mmol/l)	4.02±0.46	1.15±0.10	$p<0.001$
Fasting cholesterol (mmol/l)	5.65±0.23	4.98±0.34	n.s.
Blood pressure (mmHg):			
systolic	121±5	114±4	$p<0.08$
diastolic	80±2	72±2	$p<0.02$
Bleeding time (min.)	4.1±0.4	5.9±0.4	$p<0.01$

Fig. 5.14 Change in metabolic risk factors and blood pressure amongst diabetic Aborigines who returned from an urban existence to the traditional hunter–gatherer lifestyle. Note that the change in diet and physical activity was associated with marked improvement in all variables measured. (Modified from O'Dea K *Hypertension as an insulin-resistant disorder: genetic factors and cellular mechanisms.* Elsevier Press; Amsterdam (1991): 69–87.)

Glucose Values for Diabetes

Random sample (mmol/l)

	diabetes likely	diabetes uncertain	diabetes unlikely
venous plasma	≥11.1	5.5−<11.1	<5.5
venous blood	≥10.0	4.4−<10.0	<4.4
capillary plasma	≥12.2	5.5−<12.2	<5.5
capillary blood	≥11.1	4.4−<11.1	<4.4

Standardized OGTT (mmol/l)

		diabetes	impaired glucose tolerance
venous plasma	fasting	≥ 7.8	< 7.8
	2h	≥11.1	7.8−<11.1
venous blood	fasting	≥ 6.7	< 6.7
	2h	≥10.0	6.7−<10.0
capillary plasma	fasting	≥ 7.8	< 7.8
	2h	≥12.2	8.9−<12.2
capillary blood	fasting	≥ 6.7	< 6.7
	2h	≥11.1	7.8−<11.1

Fig. 5.15 WHO criteria for diagnosis of diabetes mellitus. Criteria are provided for diagnosis from samples taken at random, after a fast or following an OGTT. A load of 75g glucose is currently used in the OGTT as a compromise between 100g in the USA and 50g in Europe. The diagnostic criteria vary depending on whether the sample is whole blood or plasma, venous or capillary. The OGTT should be performed in the morning after an overnight fast and the subject should not be on a carbohydrate-restricted diet, but should be eating his or her usual diet.

CLINICAL ASSESSMENT OF THE DIABETIC

Diabetes is diagnosed on the basis of elevated blood or plasma glucose. The diagnosis may be confirmed by an oral glucose tolerance test on which the diagnosis of impaired glucose tolerance may also be made (Fig. 5.15). All patients on presentation should be assessed for other risk factors and possible complications. All patients should have a physical examination (including fundoscopy) (Figs 5.16–5.20). Further evidence of complications may be provided by specific investigations (Figs. 5.21–5.24).

Types of Eye Disease	
cataract	
background retinopathy	microaneurysms dot and blot haemorrhages exudates maculopathy
transitional retinopathy	intraretinal microvascular abnormalities (IRMA) soft exudates venous irregularity
proliferative retinopathy	peripheral disc rubeosis iridis (rubeotic glaucoma)
retinal vein thrombosis	

Fig. 5.16   Classification of diabetic eye disease.

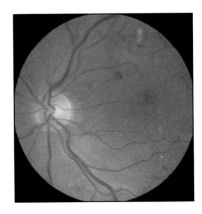

Fig. 5.17a Background retinopathy. Microaneurysms, haemorrhages and hard exudates can be seen. There is a soft exudate at 1 o'clock. (Courtesy of Mr DJ Spalton.)

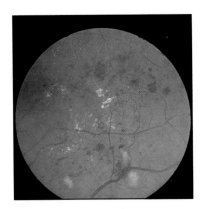

Fig. 5.17b Diabetic maculopathy. A ring of hard exudates surrounds the macula. Soft exudates, microaneurysms and deep round haemorrhages can be seen. (Courtesy of Mr J Hillman, Leeds.)

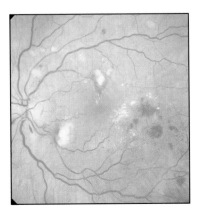

Fig. 5.17c Pre-proliferative stage of background retinopathy (transitional). This is illustrated here by large blot haemorrhages, cotton wool spots, venous irregularity and intraretinal microvascular abnormalities. (Courtesy of Mr T Metcalfe, Leeds.)

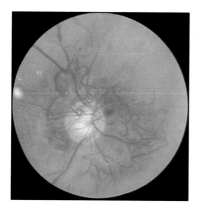

Fig. 5.17d Disc new vessels. Delicate loops of new vessels grow forward towards the vitreous (note the disc haemorrhage). They carry a serious risk of blindness if untreated. (Courtesy of Mr J Hillman, Leeds.)

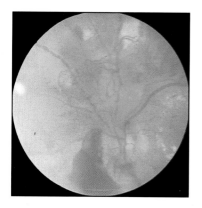

Fig. 5.17e Proliferative retinopathy. Through the vitreous, which is hazy from haemorrhage, can be seen proliferative and background changes. The bleeding site can be identified close to the disc and there is superonasal venous beading, adjacent to an area of peripheral new vessels. (Courtesy of Mr J Hillman, Leeds.)

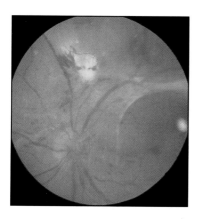

Fig. 5.17f Proliferative retinopathy. This has led to an extensive traction retinal detachment. (Courtesy of Mr J Hillman, Leeds.)

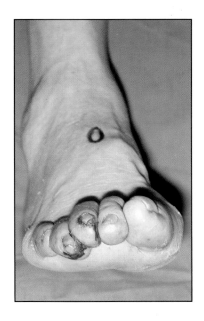

Fig. 5.18 Distal microvascular disease. In some cases of peripheral ischaemia or gangrene, the peripheral pulses may be present, implying the presence of distal microvascular disease. Ulceration may also be associated with neuropathy in the presence of foot pulses. The pulses were easily palpable (dorsalis pedis pulse marked in ink) in this patient, despite the presence of painful ischaemic toes. (Courtesy of Dr D Barnett, Leeds.)

Fig. 5.19 Dry gangrene. Ischaemic changes may culminate in dry gangrene with mummification of the dead tissue and a demarcation between the dead and viable tissues. The peripheral dead tissue may be painless and separate spontaneously. In this case, the first toe

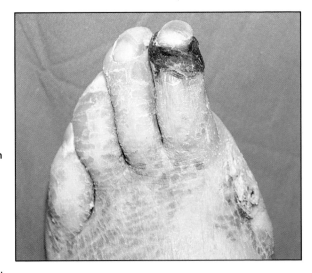

has been removed previously because of gangrene, which is now present distally in the second toe. (Courtesy of Dr D Barnett, Leeds.)

Fig. 5.20 Wet gangrene. Wet gangrene is due to ischaemia with superadded infection. A foul smell suggests the presence of anaerobes which constitutes a diabetic emergency. Urgent surgery may be required in addition to optimization of glycaemic control, antibiotics and angiography. (Courtesy of Dr D Barnett, Leeds.)

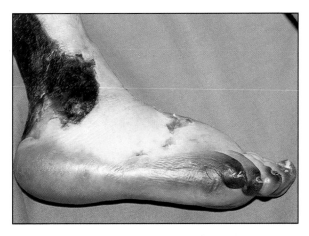

Screening for Diabetic Complications	
take history of symptoms and check for physical signs	
eye disease	visual acuity fundoscopy intraocular pressure fluorescein angiography
renal disease	albuminuria and 24h protein excretion blood pressure plasma creatinine
foot disease	inspection and clinical examination (blood and nerve supply) Doppler ultrasound blood flow nerve conduction studies
cardiac disease	chest radiography ECG
referrals to specialist clinics	ophthalmic, renal, vascular and orthopaedic

Fig. 5.21 Screening for diabetic complications.

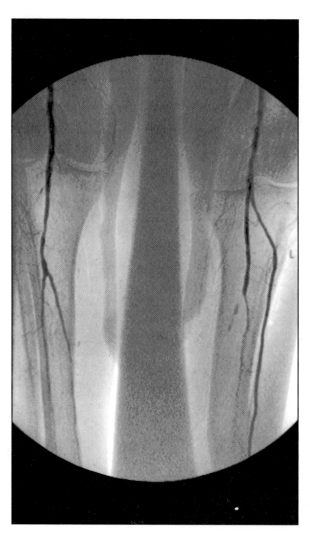

Fig. 5.22
Peripheral vascular disease. Apart from localized proximal stenoses, generally poor distal circulation is a common problem in diabetic patients. Unlike the former, poor distal circulation is more difficult to treat and may eventually necessitate local amputation. This DSA shows poor peripheral circulation past the popliteal arteries bilaterally. (Courtesy of Dr PM Chennells, Leeds.)

Fig. 5.23 Coronary angiogram. These frames are from the cine angiogram of a diabetic man with severe angina and show proximal stenoses and multiple diffuse irregularities. (a) The right coronary angiogram (right lateral projection) shows multiple critical stenoses with generalized and diffuse mural irregularity. (b) The left coronary angiogram (right anterior oblique projection) shows severe proximal stenosis and diffuse distal disease involving both the anterior descending and circumflex arteries. Diffuse disease is not amenable to surgery or angioplasty. (Courtesy of Dr HJ Bodansky, Leeds.)

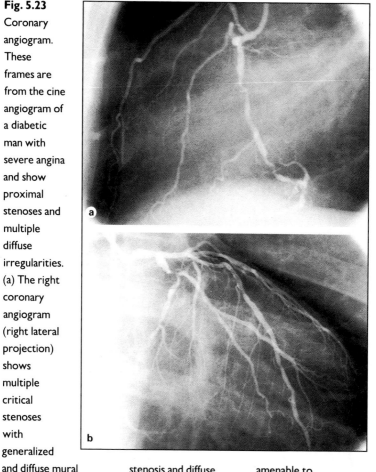

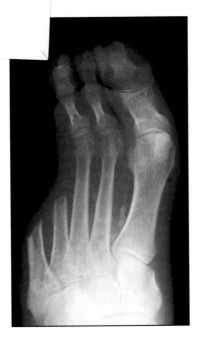

Fig. 5.24 Digital calcification in diabetes. Calcification of the digital arteries of the foot is a sign of underlying vascular disease and is seen particularly in patients with renal impairment. This patient has had amputations of the fourth and fifth toes through the metatarsals because of gangrene. (Courtesy of Dr D Barnett, Leeds.)

MANAGEMENT

The major aim of management is to prevent complications of diabetes. Management, therefore, consists of control of diabetic risk factors. These are blood glucose, lipids and blood pressure. In addition, particular attention has to be paid to associated risk factors such as smoking.

BLOOD GLUCOSE

The most frequently used method of assessing control, in the long term, is glycosylated haemoglobin measurement (normal range 4–8%) although assay of other glycosylated proteins may be used (Fig. 5.25). There have been no prospective studies demonstrating that rigid control of blood glucose is more effective than poor control. A number of retrospective studies, however, suggest that poorly controlled diabetics are at greater risk of progressive retinopathy than patients whose diabetes is well controlled (Figs 5.26 & 5.27).

The aim of treatment, therefore, should be to keep blood glucose less than 10mmol/l after meals and glycosylated haemoglobin less than 10%.

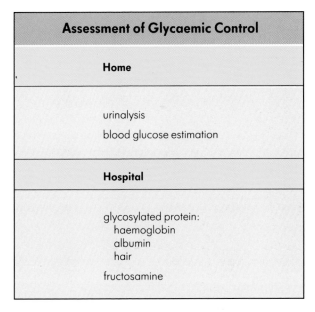

Fig. 5.25
Methods of assessment of glycaemic control.

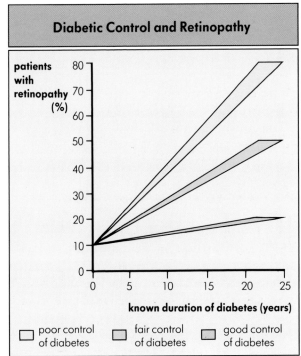

Fig. 5.26
Rate of development of retinopathy. The rate of development of complications is related to diabetic control. Grouping was based on blood glucose tests and home urinalysis. (4000 patients followed.)

This is achieved by diet and insulin in Type I diabetes and by diet alone, or diet and drugs (occasionally with insulin as well) in Type II (non-insulin-dependent diabetes). Obese patients with Type II diabetes should be maintained within 20% of ideal body weight (Fig. 5.28). Principles of

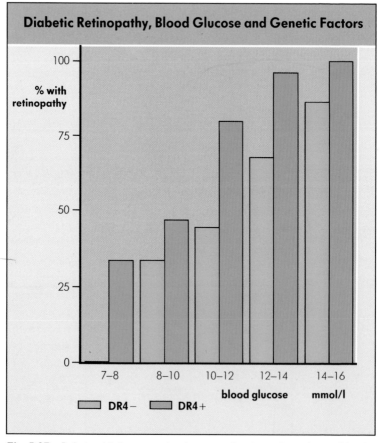

Fig. 5.27 Relationship between development of retinopathy and mean blood glucose levels in diabetic subjects. Note that the patients with a Class II antigen marker (DR4) developed retinopathy at lower blood glucose levels, indicating the role of genetic susceptibility as well as adequacy of blood glucose control. (Modified from Dornan et al. *Diabetes* 1983;**31**:226–231.)

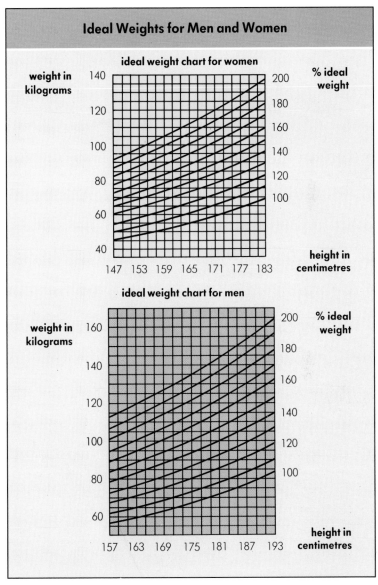

Fig. 5.28 Ideal weight charts for men and women. Data obtained from Metropolitan Life Insurance Company and presented as centiles. (Modified from Taylor KG, *Diabetes and the Heart*, Castle House Publications, Tunbridge Wells (1987).)

diet are taking regular meals containing unrefined rather than refined carbohydrate, high dietary fibre and reduced saturated fat (Fig. 5.29).

Oral hypoglycaemic agents are used in Type II diabetes, where diet is insufficient to control blood sugar. An early study with sulphonylureas (University Group Diabetes Programme) suggested that these drugs were associated with a higher mortality from coronary disease. This conclusion, however, may be due to a mismatch between different treatment groups and no further evidence in favour of this conclusion has been reported. The biguanide, metformin has the advantage that it depresses rather than stimulates appetite and is, therefore, particularly useful in obese, non-insulin-dependent subjects (Fig. 5.30). Insulin is used

Principles of Dietary Treatment
NIDDM
Obese patients: reduce weight Non-obese patients: follow diet low in refined carbohydrates (possibly increase unrefined carbohydrate)
IDDM
Total daily calorie intake takes into account: (i)   desired body weight (ii) energy expenditure (assessment of daily activities) (iii) growth (children) (iv) extra requirement, e.g. pregnancy and breast feeding Distribution of carbohydrate intake: (i)   system of food exchanges based on 10g portions (ii) individual diet plan based on personal daily routine
All patients
Avoid easily absorbed refined carbohydrates; take unrefined Emphasize dietary fibre Reduce saturated fat; substitute polyunsaturated fat Take alcohol in moderation

Fig. 5.29   Principles of dietary treatment.

in non-insulin-dependent diabetes mellitus when other method
of blood glucose have failed and particularly in patients who
weight.

In both Type I and Type II diabetes, the regimen has to be selected to
suit the lifestyle and requirements of the individual patients, bearing in
mind age, weight, work and daily routine. The dose of insulin selected is
empirical, i.e. it is that required to optimize blood glucose levels throughout the 24-hour period. It has been argued that high insulin levels in
insulin-resistant subjects are responsible for elevated blood pressure and
perhaps contribute to accelerated atheroma. This is, however, speculative
and should not play any role in clinical decisions.

Oral Hypoglycaemic Agents		
	Sulphonylureas	**Biguanides**
Mechanisms of action	enhance endogenous insulin secretion probable extra-pancreatic effects	decrease appetite reduce intestinal glucose absorption decrease gluconeogenesis increase anaerobic glycolysis increase muscle glucose uptake
Indications	diet has failed in non-obese NIDDM patient	diet has failed in NIDDM patient, particularly if obese

Fig. 5.30 Features of oral hypoglycaemic agents. If the maximal dose of one type is reached, then the other may be added if desired.

SERUM LIPIDS

Sulphonylureas probably have no effect upon serum lipids. There is some evidence that metformin may have a beneficial effect on lipid profile. Insulin plays a major role in triglyceride clearance through regulation of the enzyme lipoprotein lipase. Lipid profiles should be measured in all diabetic subjects and subjects with impaired glucose tolerance. Management is based upon the same principles as treatment of the non-diabetic subject (see Chapter 4).

HYPERTENSION

Deterioration of diabetic retinopathy, or of renal failure in patients with nephropathy, is more rapid in the presence of hypertension (Fig. 5.31). Rigorous control of blood pressure is, therefore, particularly important. Diastolic blood pressure should be maintained below 90mmHg. The normal diastolic threshold for treatment, of 100mmHg over several

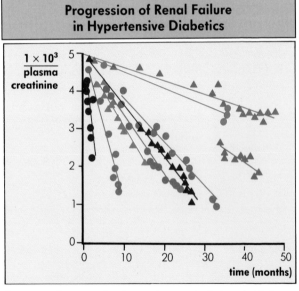

Fig. 5.31 Progression of renal failure in nine diabetic patients documented by plotting the inverse of the plasma creatinine level. Different patients have different rates of decline. This decline may be slowed by aggressive treatment of hypertension. Improving glycaemic control may reduce the microalbumin excretion rate, but probably has little or no effect on established nephropathy.

readings (see Chapter 3), should probably be reduced to 95mmHg or even 90mmHg. Systolic blood pressure, ideally, should be reduced to 140mmHg or less although in older diabetic subjects, with loss of large arterial compliance, this may be impossible to achieve in practice.

Certain classes of drugs present particular problems in diabetic subjects (Fig. 5.32). Thiazide diuretics impair glucose tolerance and therefore make glycaemic control more difficult in non-insulin-dependent diabetes mellitus. β-blockers may aggravate hypoglycaemia by inhibiting gluco-neogenesis and may impair a patient's perception of hypoglycaemic symptoms. Both thiazide diuretics and β-blockers have an adverse effect on serum lipids, although this is minimized in the case of thiazides by low dosage treatment, e.g. bendrofluazide at 2.5mg/day.

Classes of Antihypertensive Agents – Problems with Usage in Diabetics	
Thiazide diuretics	impaired glucose tolerance cholesterol ↑ triglycerides ↑ LDL-cholesterol ↑ HDL-cholesterol ↓ (minimized by usage of low dosage, e.g. bendrofluazide 2.5mg/day)
β-adrenergic receptor blockers	worsening of hypoglycaemia (decreased gluconeogenesis) (less marked with cardioselective agents) worsening of peripheral ischaemia (less marked with cardioselective agents) triglycerides ↑ HDL-cholesterol ↓ impairment of perception of hypoglycaemic symptoms
ACE inhibitors	worsening of decreased renal blood flow in renal atheroma

Fig. 5.32 Specific problems associated with different classes of antihypertensive medication in the diabetic patient. Note that other adverse reactions may occur, e.g. gout with thiazide diuretics, bronchospasm with β-blockers or cough with ACE inhibitors.

Alcohol 6

EPIDEMIOLOGY

There is an inverse relationship between coronary artery disease and alcohol intake in the general population (Fig. 6.1). This association only emerges after adjustment has been made for other risk factors since heavy alcohol intake may be a marker for an unhealthy lifestyle. Thus, heavy drinking is commonly associated with cigarette smoking, being overweight and belonging to social class IV or V. In addition, patients with established coronary artery disease are often advised to moderate their alcohol intake or abstain altogether. In this group a low alcohol intake would, therefore, be a marker for coronary artery disease. In the

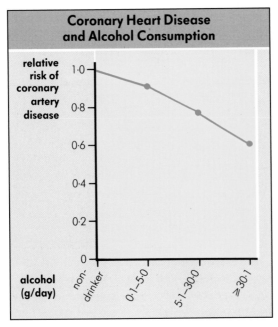

Fig. 6.1 Relative risks of alcohol consumption and coronary artery disease in 44,059 men followed for two years. (Modified from Rimm et al. Lancet 1991; **338**:464–468.)

British Regional Heart Study, for instance, when men who reported a diagnosis of cardiovascular disorders were excluded and other lifestyle factors were allowed for, there was no association between alcohol and cardiovascular mortality or coronary artery disease. However, the numbers were fairly small in this study and the much larger Health Professionals Follow-up Study of 51,529 men observed a negative association between risk of coronary artery disease and alcohol intake, which was quite independent of other lifestyle factors or the presence of known cardiovascular disease. By contrast, there is a direct relationship between alcohol intake and stroke. This extends throughout the range of drinking (Fig. 6.2).

The relationship between blood pressure and alcohol is slightly more complex (Fig. 6.3). A number of studies have shown a 'J-shaped' relationship with the lowest blood pressures in moderate drinkers. The highest blood pressures are observed in heavy drinkers.

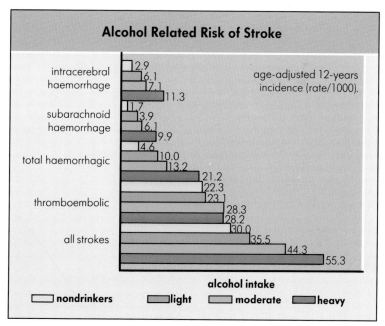

Fig. 6.2 Risk of different types of stroke in 7,878 men, free of evidence of cerebrovascular disease, followed up for 12 years. (Modified from Donahue et al. *JAMA* 1986; **255** (17):2311–2315.)

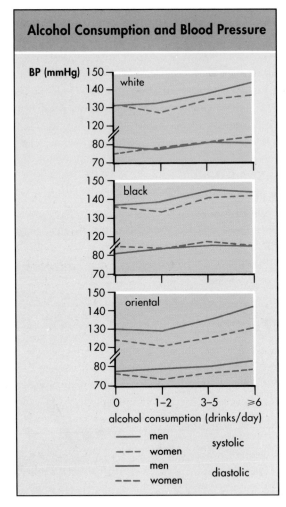

Alcohol Consumption and Blood Pressure

BP (mmHg)

white

black

oriental

alcohol consumption (drinks/day)

0 1–2 3–5 ≥6

men
women } systolic

men
women } diastolic

Fig. 6.3
Relationship of heavy alcohol consumption and blood pressure. Kaiser–Permanente questionnaire. (*New England Journal of Medicine* 1977; **296**:1194–1200.)

MECHANISMS

Increasing alcohol intake is associated with elevation of plasma HDL2 and HDL3 cholesterol, i.e. the protective fraction of cholesterol. On the other hand, some effects upon the cardiovascular system are adverse. Thus, the increase in stroke has been partially attributed to increased platelet adhesiveness, and increased osmolality and haemotocrit as a result of the inhibition of vasopressin release. Beer drinking increases calorie intake and there is an association between heavy drinking and obesity.

Acute alcohol ingestion and withdrawal of alcohol from heavy drinkers is associated with increased sympathetic nervous system activity, although there is no evidence that the autonomic nervous system mediates the sustained elevation in blood pressure in heavy drinkers.

CLINICAL FEATURES

Heavy alcohol intake is often denied by patients. Evidence for excessive drinking may be provided by relatives of the patient and a clue is often contained in the patient's occupation. Heavy drinking is particularly prevalent in those whose work involves them spending prolonged periods away from home as well as in those who work with alcoholic drinks.

Physical examination may reveal alcohol in the breath, facial telangiectasia, occasionally Dupuytren's contracture or less commonly clinical features of alcohol-induced Cushing's syndrome (Fig. 6.4). Prolonged heavy drinking may give rise to stigmata of chronic liver disease, i.e. firm, irregular, enlarged liver in the early stages and contracted liver in the advanced stages of cirrhosis. Also, 'spider naevi' in the distribution of the superior vena cava, high output state with rapid bounding pulse, loss of secondary sexual hair, foetor hepaticus and encephalopathy may present in the late stage.

Portal hypertension is indicated by splenomegaly and the presence of a caput medusae. Simple investigations often, however, provide the first indication that a patient is drinking heavily. These take the form of a slight elevation in serum transaminases and increased mean corpuscular volume on routine blood count (Fig. 6.5)

MANAGEMENT

Alcohol intake is usually classified as units. One unit is a half pint of beer, a measure of spirits or a glass of wine. The upper acceptable level for men is 21 units per week and for women, 14 units per week, since women are more sensitive to alcohol-induced liver disease.

119

The negative association between alcohol intake and coronary artery disease should not lead to acceptance of heavy drinking in patients. Thus, apart from the effect of alcohol on the liver, the predisposition to stroke, contribution of alcohol intake to obesity and the social consequences of heavy drinking underline the fact that heavy drinking should be one of the primary targets in any preventive medicine strategy. Particular attention should be paid to the possibility of heavy drinking in hypertensive patients (see Chapter 2).

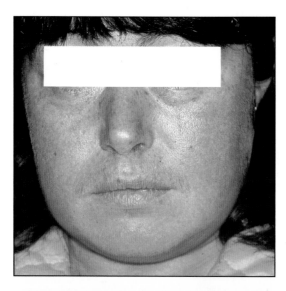

Fig. 6.4 Patient with alcohol-induced Cushing's syndrome.

Signs of Excessive Alcohol Intake	
Early	**Late**
raised transaminases	Cushingoid appearance
raised mean corpuscular volume	stigmata of liver disease
drunkenness and alcohol in breath	hepatic encephalopathy
facial telangiectasia	peripheral neuropathy
	Wernicke's encephalopathy

Fig. 6.5 Clinical and biochemical evidence of excessive alcohol intake.

Smoking   7

SMOKING AS A RISK FACTOR

Smoking, particularly cigarette smoking, is recognized as a major risk factor for angina and myocardial infarction. Taking all ages and both sexes together, the increased relative risk of coronary heart disease mortality attributable to smoking is of the order of 1.8 to 2.0. This is a much smaller increase in relative risk than that for lung cancer, but because coronary heart disease is much more common than lung cancer, the major part of excess population mortality associated with cigarette smoking is due to coronary heart disease. The relative risk of heart disease in smokers is much greater in younger patients, in particular young men. The larger the number of cigarettes smoked, the greater the increase in risk (Fig. 7.1).

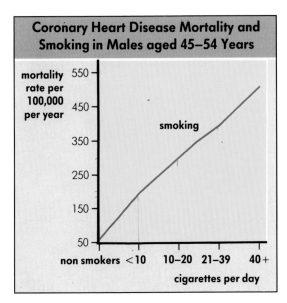

Fig. 7.1

Mortality rates per 100,000 per year from coronary heart disease, for males aged 45–54 years, as a function of the number of cigarettes smoked.

It is an important feature of smoking, as a risk factor for coronary heart disease, that it interacts very strongly with other important risk factors such as hypercholesterolaemia and hypertension (Figs 7.2 & 7.3).

POPULATION STUDIES

On a population basis, this effect is seen very strongly in countries such as China and Japan, where smoking is very prevalent, especially among the male population, but ischaemic heart disease is rare (see Chapter 10). These populations have a very low mean cholesterol concentration, and also consume large quantities of fish oil, etc. It is interesting that, as sections of these communities adopt more 'Westernized' diets, the incidence of coronary heart disease rises sharply. It is also interesting that the incidence of lung cancer is high.

RISK REVERSAL

If smoking really is a risk factor, rather than a risk marker, for coronary disease then the risk of coronary events should be reduced once the patient stops smoking. This is in fact the case (Fig. 7.4), but different

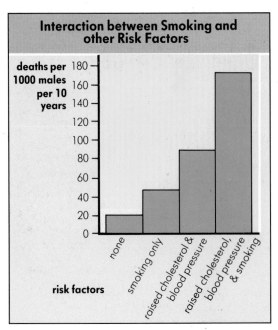

Fig. 7.2

Interaction between smoking, hypercholesterolaemia and hypertension as risk factors for coronary heart disease.

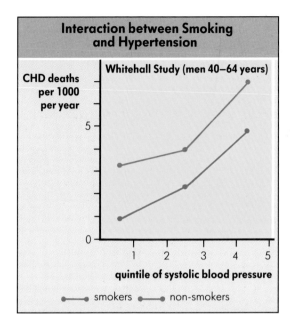

Fig. 7.3

Relationship between smoking and hypertension as risk factors for coronary heart disease.

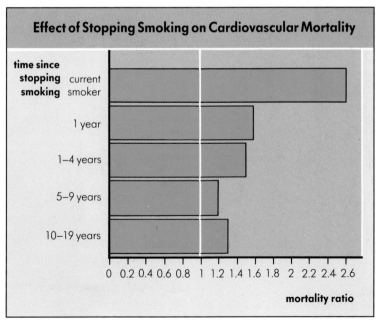

Fig. 7.4 Standardized mortality ratios for coronary heart disease for ex-smokers as a function of time since stopping.

trials have given different results concerning the rate at which it diminishes when smoking stops. This is almost certainly due to methodological differences. The decline in risk is probably biphasic, with an initial rapid

Mechanisms of Disease	
• **Via nicotine:**	increased vascular tone risk of arterial spasm increased catecholamine levels
• **Via carbon monoxide:**	impaired metabolism of vascular cells raised blood carboxyhaemoglobin content
• **Via oxygen free radicals:**	increased endothelial damage reduced plasma antioxidant levels
• **Via raised fibrinogen:**	increased thrombosis risk
• **Via altered diet:**	decreased vitamin intake

Fig. 7.5 Mechanisms by which smoking might cause coronary heart disease.

reduction in risk, perhaps due to a reduction in a tendency to vasospasm and a fall in circulating catecholamines, and a more gradual risk reduction as other factors, such as plasma fibrinogen, return to normal.

MECHANISMS OF DISEASE

The mechanism by which smoking precipitates coronary disease is uncertain, although several possible candidates have been suggested (Fig. 7.5).

Almost certainly, smoking facilitates coronary disease by a variety of different mechanisms which may be of differing importance in patients at different times. Thus, endothelial damage may, in the presence of hypercholesterolaemia, foster the development of an atheromatous plaque. Enhanced vascular tone may make the plaque more likely to rupture at a time of circulatory stress and a raised plasma fibrinogen concentration may make thrombosis on a cracked plaque more likely.

It has been suggested that the association between smoking and coronary artery disease is coincidental rather than causal, in that some, as yet unspecified, factor might simultaneously increase the risk of heart disease and produce a compulsion to smoke. However, this is hard to reconcile with the reduced heart disease risk in people who stop smoking.

It is important to remember that most UK patients are already at high risk for coronary disease because of the high population mean cholesterol concentration and, at least until recently, it has been more practicable to reduce smoking than to lower cholesterol. It is not uncommon for patients with myocardial infarction to say that they had given up smoking a few days or weeks beforehand. However, this may have been precipitated by the onset of premonitory symptoms.

Chronic smokers tend to be deficient both in ascorbic acid (vitamin C) and in certain essential fatty acids. A possible explanation is that smokers, as a group, tend to have different dietary preferences to non-smokers (Fig. 7.6).

Cessation of smoking is often accompanied by an increase in food intake and in body weight. Sometimes, this may be accompanied by a deterioration in plasma lipid profile, although this does not seem to outweigh the observed survival benefit attributed to stopping smoking.

Plasma Antioxidant Concentrations and Smoking					
	Vit A	Carotene	Vit C	Vit E	Vit E/ Cholesterol
Never smoked	2.27	0.53	40.9	23.5	3.88
Cigarette smokers	2.33	0.42	24.1	23.5	3.63
		p<0.01	p<0.001		

Fig. 7.6 Relationship between smoking and vitamin C/vitamin E concentrations in control subjects for a trial which investigated relationship between vitamin status and coronary heart disease. Cigarette smokers have strikingly lower plasma vitamin C and, less strikingly, lower carotene levels. (Modified from Reimersma RA *et al. Lancet* 1991;**337**:1–5.)

TRENDS IN SMOKING

Cigarette consumption over the past 25 years has declined dramatically amongst British doctors. It has also fallen among British males but is increasing among British females, particularly in the 15–35-year-old age group (Fig. 7.7).

Patterns of cigarette smoking in different countries vary with age, sex and social class. Smoking among women, particularly in developing countries, is increasing and this group tends to be specifically targeted by advertisers (Fig. 7.8).

Children or young adults smoking cigarettes for the first time frequently experience initial nausea, but these symptoms rarely persist. Those who enjoy cigarette smoking claim that it induces a feeling of calm combined with alertness. It is claimed that this helps the smoker to cope

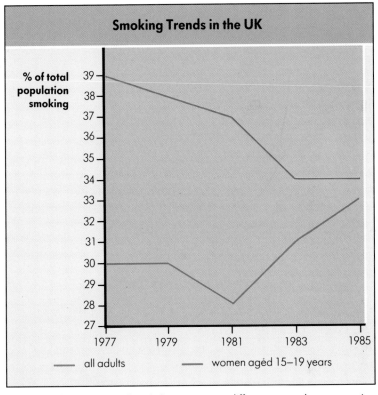

Fig. 7.7 Changes in smoking behaviour among different age and sex groups in the UK.

Smoking Trends in Different Countries	
USA	reducing in all groups
Australia	reducing in all groups
Scandinavia	reducing in all groups
UK	falling in men, increasing in young women
Italy	static in men, increasing in women
India	static in men, increasing in women

Fig. 7.8 Changes in smoking patterns in different countries.

127

with stress. Cigarette consumption tends to increase during periods of stress or emotional arousal.

Smoking habits differ from individual to individual. Some remain light or occasional smokers, whereas others experience a progressive compulsion to increase cigarette consumption. Similarly, some individuals find it easy to stop smoking, whereas others find it extremely difficult, even in the presence of obvious and acknowledged evidence of damage to health. At least, in a proportion of smokers, smoking appears to have the properties of a classical addictive drug, namely, a tendency to increase the dose, intense craving and a withdrawal syndrome characterized by anxiety, irritability, and sometimes physical symptoms such as tremor. The reasons for the apparent difference, in dependence and addictive capacity between individuals, are not well understood.

ATTITUDES TOWARDS SMOKING

Public health policy on smoking, in those countries which have adopted such a policy, has aimed at persuasion rather than prohibition. In the UK there are restrictions on the nature of tobacco advertisements and the media which can be used. Advertisements for tobacco products carry "Government Health Warnings". Tobacco products are subject to high taxation, although this is potentially counterproductive, as the tax income comes to be regarded as indispensable (Fig. 7.9).

Persuasion strategies tend to be most effective in groups where the harmful consequences of smoking can most readily be perceived or where there is peer group pressure (Fig. 7.10). Smoking is more prevalent, and stopping smoking more difficult, in populations under physical or emotional stress, such as intensive care nurses.

Individual patients tend to be most successful at stopping smoking if there is a powerful motivational event (Fig. 7.11). This could be a myocardial infarction or bypass surgery, either in the patient or in a close relative. Alternatively, there may be others in the family or peer group, who are either non-smokers or who have given up smoking, able to give the patient adequate medical and social support. Some patients find a nicotine substitute, such as nicotine impregnated chewing gum, helpful as an adjunct to supervision and counselling. Others may choose different forms of displacement activity.

128

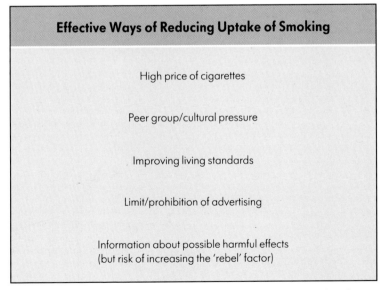

UK/EEC Attitudes to Tobacco	
Public information on smoking hazards:	Yes
'Punitive' taxation: (taxation increases, but whether this is an increase in real terms is debatable)	?
Restrictions on advertising:	Yes
Prohibition of advertising:	No
Ban on smoking in public places/transport	Yes, variable
EEC support for tobacco growers	Yes

Fig. 7.9 Summary of public health policy on smoking in the UK and EEC.

Effective Ways of Reducing Uptake of Smoking
High price of cigarettes
Peer group/cultural pressure
Improving living standards
Limit/prohibition of advertising
Information about possible harmful effects (but risk of increasing the 'rebel' factor)

Fig. 7.10 Factors contributing to individual success in reducing uptake of smoking.

129

Effective Ways of Stopping Smoking	
Major life event	(e.g. heart attack)
Peer group	family support (e.g. husband & wife stop together)
Stress reduction	relief of symptoms
Diversion of interests	(e.g. new hobby)
Avoidance of secondary effects	(e.g. weight gain)

Fig. 7.11 Factors contributing to individual success in stopping smoking.

Other Metabolic Risk Markers and Risk Factors

8

URIC ACID

Uric acid is a product of the oxidation of xanthine by xanthine oxidase, a reaction which produces oxygen free radicals. The relevance of this, if any, to clinical coronary disease is uncertain. However, elevated plasma uric acid concentrations have been associated, epidemiologically, with an increased risk of coronary artery disease (Fig. 8.1). This association is independent of renal function and the mechanism of the link is unclear.

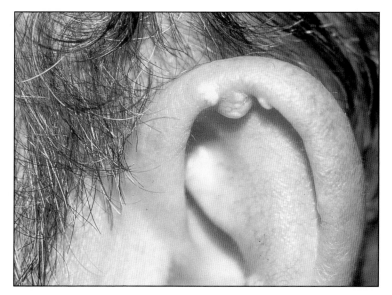

Fig. 8.1 Gouty tophus. Hyperuricaemia is a marker for ischaemic heart disease at much lower concentrations than those associated with clinical gout. (By courtesy of Dr Anthony du Vivier.)

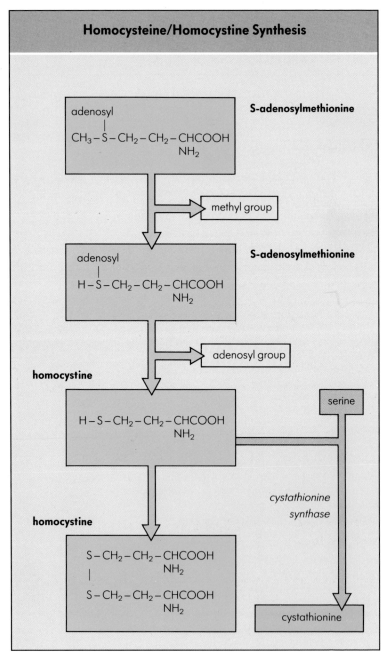

Fig. 8.2 Structures and synthesis of homocysteine and homocystine.

Uric acid is mainly produced as a breakdown product of nucleic acids and may be increased in people whose diet is rich in meat. Increased plasma uric acid levels are also associated with increased tissue turnover and with conditions leading to a polymorph leukocytosis. It has also been suggested that uric acid is a marker for increased endothelial cell damage.

HOMOCYSTINE

Homocystinuria/homocysteinaemia is an inborn error of metabolism characterized by the presence of excessive quantities of homocystine in the urine and homocysteine in the blood. Homocysteine is produced from the dietary amino acid methionine (Fig. 8.2) and is an intermediate in the production of cystathionine, which helps protect cells from oxidative damage. A deficiency of cystathionine synthase leads to an excess of homocysteine, molecules of which combine to form homocystine.

In its homozygous form it is associated with learning difficulties and with an increased incidence of vascular thrombosis. This has been associated with an increased rate of damage to vascular endothelial cells *in vivo*. Patients are often fair-skinned and have fair hair.

This condition is very rare but recently a number of studies have shown a correlation between mildly elevated plasma homocysteine concentrations and coronary artery disease in a much wider section of the community. Sometimes, plasma homocysteine levels are normal but rise excessively after a test meal containing the amino acid methionine. The overall significance of mild homocysteinaemia as a cause of coronary artery disease is at present uncertain.

VITAMIN C (ASCORBIC ACID) AND VITAMIN E (TOCOPHEROL)

Both ascorbic acid and tocopherol are biological antioxidants. Many components of body tissues are susceptible to auto-oxidation. This includes low density lipoprotein, either in the plasma or after its uptake into the vessel wall. Oxidized low density lipoprotein is capable of attracting macrophages, and may initiate inflammatory reactions which contribute to the growth and sometimes to the instability of atheromatous plaques (Fig. 8.3).

133

Patients who have had a myocardial infarction tend to have lower plasma concentrations of water-soluble ascorbic acid and lower adipose tissue concentrations of fat-soluble tocopherol (Fig. 8.4). Interestingly, this deficiency also correlates with smoking, and it has been suggested that smokers deliberately consume less of the foods containing these anti-oxidant substances.

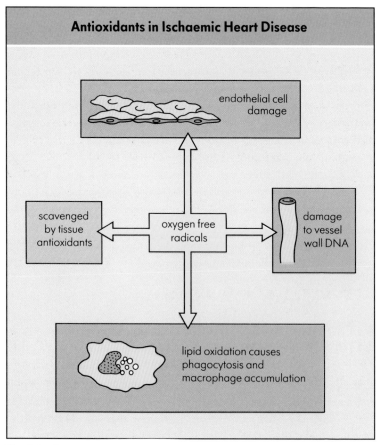

Fig. 8.3 Possible mechanism by which lack of biological antioxidants can produce ischaemic heart disease.

Plasma Antioxidants in Angina Patients		
	Controls	**Cases**
Vitamin A (mol/l)	2.32	2.29 ns
Carotene (mol/l)	0.49	0.30 <0.001
Vitamin C (mol/l)	35.3	28.1 <0.01
Vitamin E (mol/l)	24.0	22.7 ns
Vitamin E/cholesterol (mol/mmol)	3.86	3.66 <0.01

Fig. 8.4 Concentrations of vitamin C and vitamin E in plasma from patients with and without clinical ischaemic heart disease. The angina cases had significantly lower concentrations of carotene, vitamin C, and a lower vitamin E/cholesterol ratio. (Modified from Reimersma RA *et al. Lancet* 1991;**337**:1–5.)

ESSENTIAL FATTY ACIDS

Certain polyunsaturated fatty acids are called 'essential' because they cannot be synthesized *de novo* within the body (Fig. 8.5). Essential fatty acids are stored in fat tissue and also form a part of cell membranes. Their proportion may affect membrane fluidity, they can be metabolized into pharmacologically active substances, such as the thromboxanes and prostacyclins and they affect the susceptibility of cell membranes to auto-oxidation. The beneficial effects of diets rich in fish oil on coronary artery disease have been attributed to the presence of eicosopentanoic acid, which tends to depress platelet procoagulant activity.

135

Essential Fatty Acids

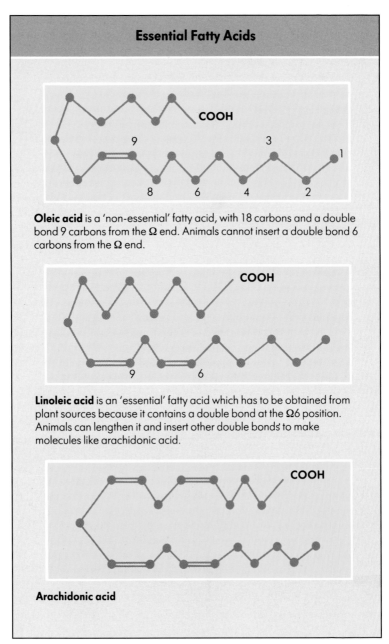

Oleic acid is a 'non-essential' fatty acid, with 18 carbons and a double bond 9 carbons from the Ω end. Animals cannot insert a double bond 6 carbons from the Ω end.

Linoleic acid is an 'essential' fatty acid which has to be obtained from plant sources because it contains a double bond at the Ω6 position. Animals can lengthen it and insert other double bonds to make molecules like arachidonic acid.

Arachidonic acid

Fig. 8.5   The need for 'essential' fatty acids is created by the body's inability to insert a double bond at the Ω 6 position.

Haematological Factors and Coronary Heart Disease   9

CORONARY THROMBOSIS

The interaction between blood coagulation and disease of the blood vessel wall in producing coronary heart disease has been recognized for over a century. It can take several forms. In myocardial infarction (Fig. 9.1) atheromatous plaque narrows the vessel and at the same time exposes material which promotes blood clotting. The resulting thrombus completely blocks the vessel and leads to death of the heart muscle downstream.

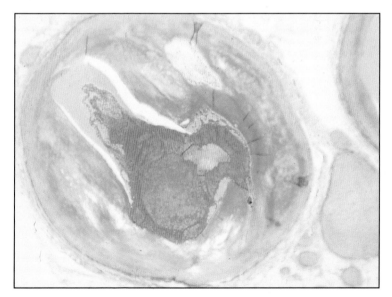

Fig. 9.1 Photomicrograph of the coronary artery from a patient with myocardial infarction to show a thrombus. (Courtesy of Prof M.J. Davies.)

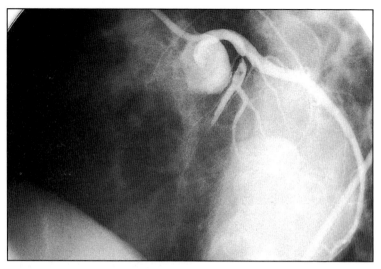

Fig. 9.2 Coronary angiogram from a patient with unstable angina showing a thrombus in the coronary lumen.

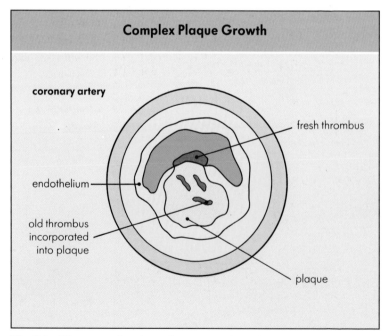

Fig. 9.3 Diagram to show how plaque grows through cycles of cracking and thrombosis.

138

In unstable angina (Fig. 9.2) a thrombus forms which is large enough to narrow the vessel and cause symptoms but not big enough to block it completely. Finally, there is evidence that some complex atheromatous plaques have been through many cycles of growth, cracking, thrombosis and healing without the vessel ever becoming completely blocked (Fig. 9.3).

HAEMATOLOGICAL MEASUREMENTS

There are a large number of haematological measurements which have been shown to correlate either with the presence of coronary artery disease or with the risk of suffering a myocardial infarct (Fig. 9.4). For some, we can advance a plausible mechanism. For others, we simply have to accept an epidemiological linkage, which may or may not be causal.

Haematological Risk Factors
Cellular factors
Polycythaemia (high red cell count) Polymorph leukocytosis (high white cell count) Thrombocytosis (high platelet count) Large volume platelets
Coagulation factors
High fibrinogen High factor VII Low or high antithrombin III
Fibrinolytic system
Low or high plasminogen activator (in plasma) High plasminogen activator inhibitor

Fig. 9.4
Haematological factors shown to correlate with risk of myocardial infarction or ischaemic heart disease.

RED CELLS

There is an epidemiological correlation, particularly in men, between an increased red cell count, or raised haemoglobin level, and risk of coronary artery disease and myocardial infarction. The mechanism is unclear. Smokers tend to have higher red blood cell counts than non-smokers, also a high red blood cell count could be an index of dehydration which might precipitate thrombosis.

LEUKOCYTOSIS

There is an epidemiological correlation between a high white blood cell count and risk of coronary artery disease (Fig. 9.5). Again, the mechanism is speculative. A raised leukocyte count may reflect ongoing tissue, including vascular, damage. Polymorphonuclear leukocytes produce

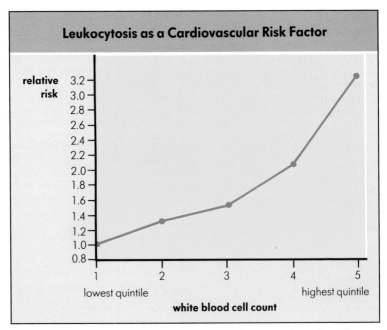

Fig. 9.5 Relative risk of a major ischaemic heart disease incident, plotted against quintile of white blood cell count. (Modified from Yarnell JWG et al. *Circulation* 1991; **83**:836–44.)

oxygen-centred free radicals which injure vascular endothelium. A high leukocyte count is sometimes associated with raised plasma uric acid, which is also a known risk marker for coronary artery disease.

PLATELETS

A markedly raised platelet count, thrombocytosis, is sometimes associated with an increased risk of vascular thrombosis. Many attempts have been made to link various measures of platelet function with coronary artery disease risk but these tests tend to be technically difficult, hard to repeat and so far of little practical value in identifying high risk individuals. An exception may be the measurement of platelet size (Fig. 9.6) which does seem to be positively correlated with myocardial infarct risk. The mechanism is unknown.

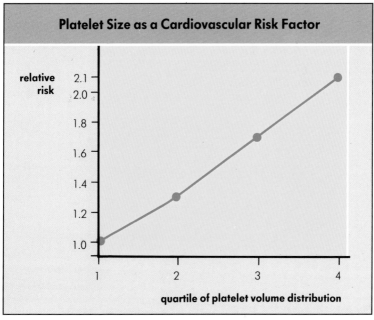

Fig. 9.6 Relationship between platelet size and risk of myocardial infarction. (Modified from Martin JF, Bath PMW & Burr ML, *Lancet* 1991; **338**:1409–1411.)

FIBRINOGEN

Plasma fibrinogen is the source of fibrin, the main protein involved in forming the structure of a thrombus. As expected, there is a positive correlation between plasma fibrinogen concentration and risk of myocardial infarction. Factors which raise plasma fibrinogen include smoking and tissue damage (fibrinogen is one of a group of proteins called acute phase reactants because their plasma concentration tends to increase after injury of any sort). There is an increased risk of myocardial infarction during cold weather which correlates with increased plasma fibrinogen concentration under these conditions (Fig. 9.7). There is also a correlation between smoking and increased plasminogen concentration.

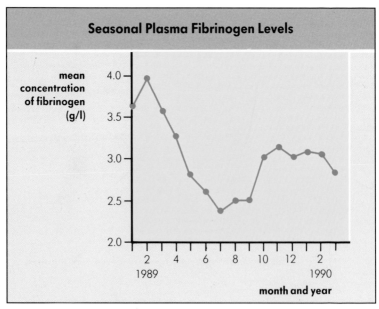

Fig. 9.7 Changes in plasma fibrinogen concentration with ambient temperature. (Modified from Stout RW & Crawford L, *Lancet* 1991; **338**:9–13.)

FACTOR VII

Factor VII is one of the blood coagulation factors which form part of the cascade eventually ending in the activation of prothrombin to thrombin and thus, the conversion of fibrinogen to fibrin. Epidemiologically, there is a strong correlation between raised factor VII levels and risk of myocardial infarction (Fig. 9.8).

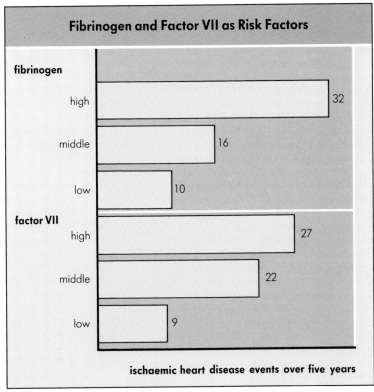

Fig. 9.8 Relationship of plasma fibrinogen concentration and factor VII concentration to risk of cardiac events. Deaths and non-fatal myocardial infarctions over a five-year period. (Modified from Meade TW *et al. Lancet* 1986; ii:533–537.)

ANTITHROMBIN III

Antithrombin III is a plasma protein which tends to check the action of the procoagulant thrombin. The relationship between plasma antithrombin III concentration and coronary disease is interesting because it seems that both very low and very high antithrombin III levels are associated with an increased risk of coronary thrombosis (Fig. 9.9). The reason for this is unclear. It may be that very high antithrombin III levels are an adaptive response to increased deactivation of the coagulant by some other mechanism.

PLASMA FIBRINOLYTIC ACTIVITY

Plasma fibrinolytic activity is the result of a balance between tissue plasminogen activator (t-pa), which is released from endothelium and promotes fibrinolysis, and plasminogen activator inhibitor, also released from endothelial cells, which inactivates tissue plasminogen activator.

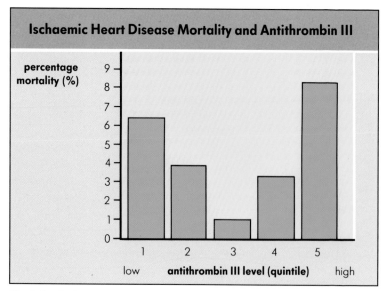

Fig. 9.9 Both very high and very low antithrombin III levels correlate with increased risk of ischaemic heart disease. (Modified from Meade TW *et al. Lancet* 1991; **338**:850–851.)

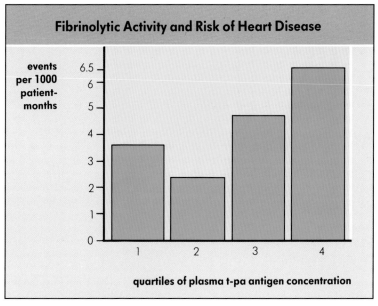

Fig. 9.10   Interrelation between plasma fibrinolytic activity (plasma t-pa antigen concentration) and incidence of coronary ischaemic events. (Modified from Jansson, Nilsson & Olofsson, *Eur Heart J* 1991; **12**:157–162.)

There is a marked diurnal variation in plasma fibrinolytic activity which reflects changes in tissue plasminogen activator and inhibitor levels. In general, these levels tend to be lowest at night and rise in the morning. They are increased by vigorous physical activity but there is often then a rebound period of reduced plasma fibrinolytic activity in the early hours of the morning, with a predilection for myocardial infarction to occur between breakfast time and midday, but there are other possible reasons for this (Fig. 9.10).

In young European men with first myocardial infarcts, Hamsten has shown a relative deficiency of plasma fibrinolytic activity. This seems to be independent of lipid concentrations, although raised plasma trigly-cerides can also inhibit plasma fibrinolytic activity. Interestingly, plasma fibrinolytic activity is increased in South Asians who, otherwise, tend to have a rather increased prevalence of coronary artery disease. Both the mechanism and the significance of this are unclear.

145

Target Organ Damage   *10*

CORONARY ARTERY DISEASE

CLINICAL FEATURES
The three principal clinical manifestations of coronary artery disease are:
- myocardial infarction
- angina pectoris
- cardiac failure.

Myocardial infarction may be manifest, clinically, as an episode of severe chest pain and collapse, but is sometimes clinically silent. Electrocardiographic features of infarction (Fig. 10.1) may be found in patients

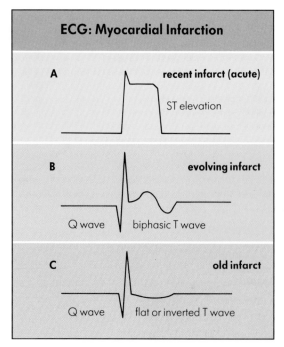

ECG: Myocardial Infarction

A — recent infarct (acute)
ST elevation

B — evolving infarct
Q wave — biphasic T wave

C — old infarct
Q wave — flat or inverted T wave

Fig. 10.1 The electrocardiographic features of myocardial infarction: (A) acute infarct with ST segment elevation; (B) evolving infarct with Q wave and biphasic T wave; (C) old infarct with Q wave and flat T wave.

who deny ever having had symptoms. The chest radiograph is usually unhelpful, but echocardiographic demonstration of a hypokinetic or akinetic ventricular segment can corroborate the electrocardiographic findings.

Angina pectoris is essentially a clinical diagnosis, but treadmill exercise testing helps confirm the diagnosis and evaluate severity. Coronary arteriography (Fig. 10.2) demonstrates the stenoses causing symptoms and may precede coronary angioplasty or bypass grafting.

The attribution of cardiac failure to coronary artery disease is straight-forward if it occurs in the aftermath of a myocardial infarct, but otherwise it can be difficult, short of coronary angiography, to distinguish between heart failure due to coronary artery disease and heart failure which is due to a cardiomyopathy.

EPIDEMIOLOGY

Patients with angina pectoris are at increased risk of cardiovascular death or myocardial infarction. Despite this they actually contribute only about 20% of the total population suffering these events. Longitudinal studies of the natural history of coronary artery stenoses indicate that different stenoses progress at different rates, and a new infarct in a patient who has previously had coronary arteriography frequently originates at a point where the previous images show no detectable lesion.

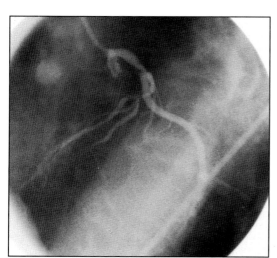

Fig. 10.2
Coronary arteriogram showing severe coronary artery disease, including left main coronary artery stenosis.

RISK FACTORS AND PROGNOSIS

Any patient with one or more manifestations of coronary artery disease is at increased risk of cardiovascular mortality compared to the general population.

Prognosis after myocardial infarction is principally determined by:
- age of the patient, younger better than older
- site of the infarct, inferior better than anterior
- left ventricular ejection fraction
- the presence of residual angina.

Patients with a left ventricular ejection fraction of less than 20% have a one-year mortality of the order of 20%. Residual angina and/or a positive exercise test are markers for an increased risk of recurrent infarction, but this can be modified by intervention. Risk factors such as hypercholesterolaemia, smoking and hypertension have a similar proportionate effect on cardiovascular risk after a myocardial infarct to that which they have in a 'normal' population, although the absolute risk is increased. Secondary prevention is therefore more cost effective than primary prevention.

The risk of death or non-fatal myocardial infarction in a patient with angina depends on:
- age of the patient
- time since the onset of angina (recent onset, or recently worsening angina, has a poorer prognosis)
- left ventricular function
- exercise tolerance (taking into account symptoms, ECG changes and a fall in BP with increasing exercise)
- coronary lesions (number and distribution).

The latter two points are to some extent independent predictors of outcome, and ideally both should be known to give an accurate prognosis. In practice, however, restricted resources mean that exercise testing is predominantly used as a screen to pick out 'high risk' patients for coronary angiography. After angiography, patients with left main coronary artery stenosis, three vessel disease (stenoses affecting left anterior descending and circumflex branches of the left, and also the right, coronary artery) or two vessel disease involving the proximal left anterior descending coronary artery are usually recommended to have coronary bypass surgery. This has been shown to reduce their mortality risk.

The prognosis in patients with cardiac failure caused by ischaemic heart disease is, like that in any form of cardiac failure, poor with mortality rates of up to 25% per year for severely symptomatic and 10% per year for mildly symptomatic patients.

MANAGEMENT
Myocardial Infarction
Myocardial infarction is best treated with thrombolytic therapy and aspirin (Fig. 10.3). The main period of risk for fatal arrhythmias is within the first 24 hours. Thrombolytic therapy not only improves survival but

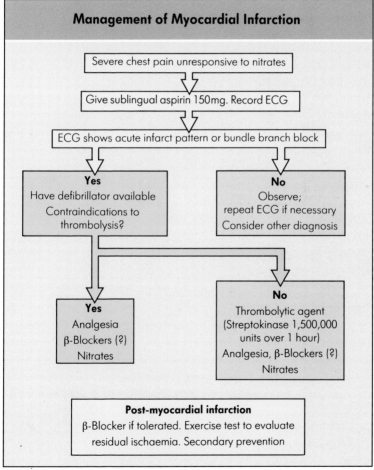

Fig. 10.3 Flow chart for the immediate management of myocardial infarction.

also reduces the proportion of surviving patients with very poor left ventricular function. There is no consensus on the length of time for which aspirin should continue to be taken; many patients do so indefinitely. β-Adrenoceptor antagonists such as timolol have been shown to improve one-year survival after myocardial infarction. Again, there is no consensus as to whether there is benefit from continuing their use after this time. Long-term β-blockade may make control of plasma lipids more difficult.

Angiotensin converting enzyme inhibitors such as enalapril have been shown to help in the prevention of 'infarct expansion', progressive dilatation of the left ventricle, particularly in patients who have had an anterior infarct. Their effect on overall mortality has not yet been assessed. Post-infarct exercise testing helps to identify patients with residual ischaemia, who may benefit from revascularization by angioplasty or coronary bypass grafting.

Angina

Aspirin has been shown to improve the chances of infarct-free survival in patients who have recovered from unstable angina and this has been extended to apply to all angina patients. There is evidence that life expectancy for angina patients has improved markedly over the period since the introduction of modern antianginal medication. However, despite β-adrenoceptor antagonists, calcium antagonists and long-acting nitrates all being effective in relieving symptoms, there is no direct evidence from controlled trials to indicate the superiority of one medication over another.

Coronary Bypass Grafting

This has been shown to improve survival, compared to 'best medical treatment', in patients with left main coronary artery stenosis, three vessel disease or two vessel disease involving the left anterior descending coronary artery. The proportionate benefit is greater in patients with impaired left ventricular function, although the initial operative mortality is higher.

Coronary Angioplasty

This may reduce the risk of subsequent myocardial infarction in patients who present with unstable angina (Figs 10.4 & 10.5), however, there is no evidence that it affects the infarct-free survival rate in patients with stable angina. It is contraindicated in left main coronary artery stenosis and experience is too limited for adequate comparison with coronary bypass grafting in the situations where the latter is known to improve survival.

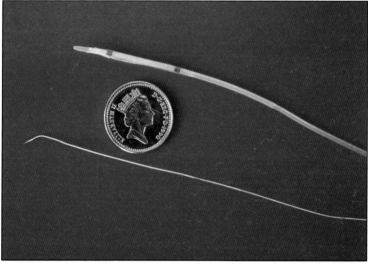

Fig. 10.4   Balloon angioplasty catheter for coronary angioplasty. The fine, gold plated guidewire is passed across the stenosis and used to guide the balloon into position.

Comparisons with medical therapy have been few, but in one recent study angioplasty gave better symptomatic relief at six months, at the cost of an increased risk of emergency coronary bypass grafting and a slightly increased risk of myocardial infarction and mortality.

Secondary prevention measures aimed at stopping smoking, correcting hypertension and plasma lipid abnormalities are particularly worthwhile and important in patients who have already suffered a myocardial infarction or who have angina. Recent evidence suggests that rigorous control of plasma cholesterol not only improves prognosis but also helps to alleviate symptoms.

151

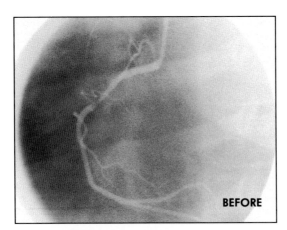

Fig. 10.5 Pre-
and post-
angioplasty
arteriograms
showing
disappearance of
the stenosis after
successful
angioplasty.

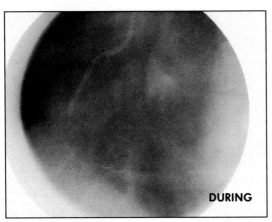

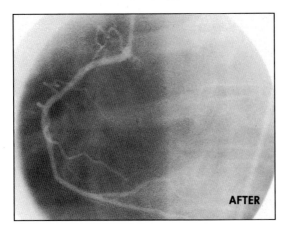

PERIPHERAL VASCULAR DISEASE AND TRANSIENT ISCHAEMIC ATTACKS

CLINICAL FEATURES OF PERIPHERAL VASCULAR DISEASE

Peripheral vascular disease is a shorthand term for arterial disease occurring outside the heart or the cranium. Its two principal manifestations are arterial stenoses and aneurysms.

The commonest clinical presentation resulting from arterial stenosis is intermittent claudication. This is pain and stiffness in the leg brought on by walking, relieved by rest and resulting from arterial obstruction, usually at the level of the iliac or femoral artery. Analogous symptoms may affect the upper limbs but are much less common. The diagnosis is supported by the absence or weakness of peripheral pulses, and confirmed by ultrasound studies or angiography (Fig. 10.6). In diabetics, intermittent claudication is less common as a presenting symptom. Patients commonly present with indolent infection and gangrene.

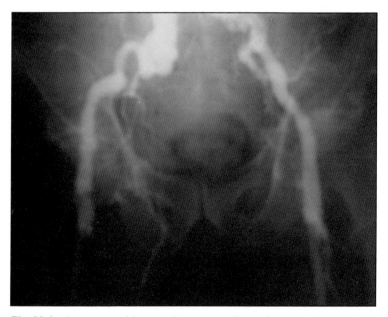

Fig. 10.6 Angiogram of iliac vessels in a man suffering from intermittent claudication showing grossly atheromatous, tortuous iliac arteries. (Courtesy of Dr R. Keal.)

153

The commonest site for aneurysm formation is in the abdominal aorta. Rupture of an aneurysm causes pain and may lead to death from internal bleeding, but many aneurysms are detected as chance findings on abdominal examination.

The risk factors for peripheral vascular disease tend to parallel those for coronary artery disease, with smoking and hypertriglyceridaemia being even more prominent. There is evidence for a genetic component in abdominal aortic aneurysm.

The principal cause of mortality in patients with peripheral vascular disease is in fact coronary artery disease. Angiographic studies demonstrate significant coronary artery stenoses in over 90% of patients with peripheral vascular disease.

MANAGEMENT OF PERIPHERAL VASCULAR DISEASE

Possible management strategies are summarized in Figure 10.7. Reconstructive vascular surgery or percutaneous angioplasty can be used to treat arterial stenoses. However, the risk of amputation if the procedure should fail and the element of risk in anaesthesia means that these procedures are usually reserved for patients with severe symptoms, or in whom the viability of the limb is in jeopardy. Peripheral vasodilators are of no proven benefit. Aspirin almost certainly helps reduce the risk of cardiovascular mortality. Stopping smoking helps limb perfusion and may improve limb viability. Reducing plasma cholesterol concentration has been shown to cause regression in iliac artery stenoses, and probably helps overall outcome. There is consensus that elective operation on abdominal aortic aneurysms improves survival, but some controversy over the precise size at which surgery should be undertaken. Most aneurysms larger than 6cm should certainly be considered for surgery.

CAROTID ARTERY DISEASE AND CEREBRAL ISCHAEMIA

Carotid artery stenosis is a variant of peripheral vascular disease which causes specific symptoms because of the role of the internal carotid artery in supplying blood to the cerebral hemispheres. The proximal part of the internal carotid artery is one of the sites of predilection for atheroma. Symptoms may be caused either by the occlusion or severe stenosis of the artery reducing blood supply to the brain, or by small portions of thrombus breaking off and causing cerebral embolism.

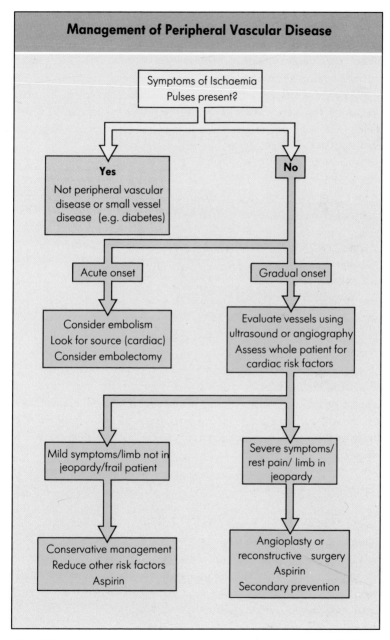

Fig. 10.7 Summary of management strategies for patients with peripheral arterial disease.

Transient ischaemic attacks, defined as transient episodes of focal impairment of neurological function with functional recovery within 24 hours, are a common clinical manifestation of these emboli. A carotid territory transient ischaemic attack might, for example, manifest itself as transient loss of speech and/or clumsiness in hand movement. There is frequently, but not invariably, a murmur or bruit over the affected vessel. Duplex ultrasound scanning (Fig. 10.8) is the most useful diagnostic technique, followed if appropriate by angiography.

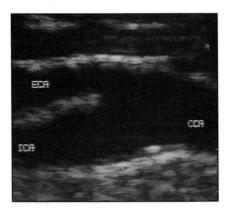

Fig. 10.8 Ultrasound image of the carotid bifurcation. Ultrasound imaging is the method of choice for detecting carotid stenosis. (Courtesy of Mr T. Hartshorne.)

MANAGEMENT OF TRANSIENT ISCHAEMIC ATTACKS

Transient ischaemic attacks are important both as a warning of an increased risk of stroke and as an indicator of generalized vascular disease. In patients with severe carotid stenosis, long term prognosis is improved by carotid endarterectomy, at the cost of slightly increased stroke risk at the time of operation. For patients with mild carotid stenosis, endarterectomy is not indicated, and anti-platelet therapy with aspirin is advised.

The optimum management of moderate carotid stenosis is still under investigation. As with other forms of peripheral vascular disease, a substantial proportion of patients presenting with transient ischaemic attacks will ultimately die of ischaemic heart disease, and secondary prevention measures as discussed previously are important. The management options are summarized in Figure 10.9.

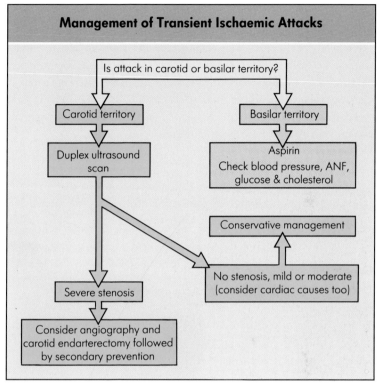

Management of Transient Ischaemic Attacks

Is attack in carotid or basilar territory?

Carotid territory

Basilar territory

Duplex ultrasound scan

Aspirin
Check blood pressure, ANF, glucose & cholesterol

Conservative management

No stenosis, mild or moderate (consider cardiac causes too)

Severe stenosis

Consider angiography and carotid endarterectomy followed by secondary prevention

Fig. 10.9 Summary of management options for patients with transient ischaemic attacks.

LEFT VENTRICULAR HYPERTROPHY

CLINICAL FEATURES

Enlargement of the cavities of the heart (dilatation) or increase in mass of the heart wall muscle (hypertrophy), may result from either intrinsic cardiac disease or an increase in work carried out by the heart. Increased left ventricular mass can, therefore, under some circumstances by physiological, in trained athletes for instance. Where dilatation or hypertrophy occur as a consequence of disease, however, they are associated with a poorer prognosis.

157

Clinically, left ventricular enlargement gives rise to displacement of the apex beat which is usually localized, forceful and heaving. In right ventricular enlargement the apex beat is not displaced but is usually tapping in quality and right ventricular contraction is felt as a left parasternal heave. Radiologically, marked cardiac enlargement is seen as increased ratio of cardiac to thoracic diameter (Fig. 10.10). Both clinical and radiological diagnoses are, however, very insensitive and abnormalities are only observed in advanced disease.

Ventricular hypertrophy may be more precisely identified by electrocardiography and echocardiography. The detection of right ventricular hypertrophy by these techniques is of importance only in relation to the primary cause, for example cor pulmonale. However, great interest has recently been attached to left ventricular hypertrophy as an independent risk factor.

Electrocardiography

Electrocardiographically, left ventricular hypertrophy is detected by:

- left axis deviation
- deep S waves in V1 to V3 and tall R waves in V4 to V6, so that the sum of the two exceeds 35mm

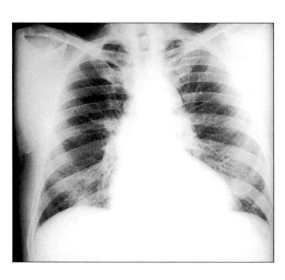

Fig. 10.10
Cardiac enlargement due to left ventricular hypertrophy in a hypertensive patient.

- inverted T waves and ST depression in lead V1, aVL and lateral chest leads in more advanced left ventricular hypertrophy (Fig. 10.11).

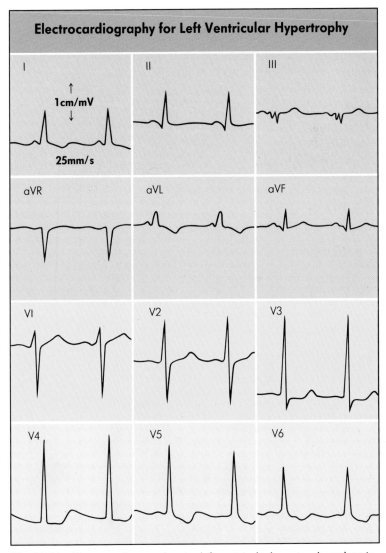

Electrocardiography for Left Ventricular Hypertrophy

Fig. 10.11 Electrocardiogram showing left ventricular hypertrophy and strain pattern. Note the deep S waves in lead V1 and tall QRS waves in leads V4 and V5 with ST depression in leads V4 to V6.

Although electrocardiography is more sensitive than a plain chest film, many patients with significant left ventricular hypertrophy will be missed if only ECG criteria are used.

Echocardiography

Echocardiography is the test of choice for detecting left ventricular hypertrophy. For most patients M mode echocardiography is sufficient although, where the geometry of the left ventricle is distorted, for example by an aneurysm, two dimensional echocardiography is preferable (Fig. 10.12). Magnetic resonance imaging has yet to enter routine clinical practice.

EPIDEMIOLOGY

In most cases electrocardiographic or echocardiographic left ventricular hypertrophy is associated with high blood pressure. In only a minority of patients is left ventricular hypertrophy associated with aortic stenosis, ischaemic heart disease or hypertrophic cardiomyopathy for instance.

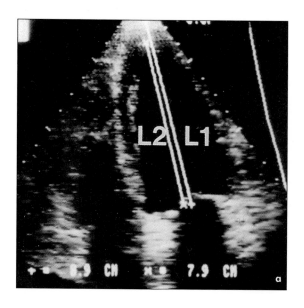

Studies of the prognosis of left ventricular hypertrophy have, therefore, only been carried out in patients with elevated blood pressure.

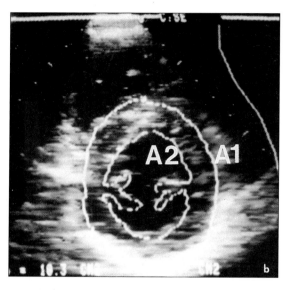

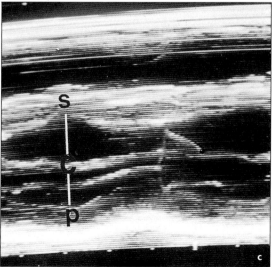

Fig. 10.12
(a) The two-dimensional echocardiographic technique showing measurements of left ventricular lengths (L1 & L2).
(b) Short axis view of heart and the planimetered epicardial (A1) and endocardial (A2) areas.
(c) M mode technique for the determination of left ventricular mass.

Electrocardiographic left ventricular hypertrophy has been reported in 3–8% of unselected hypertensive patients whilst echocardiographic left ventricular hypertrophy has been reported in 12–30% of hypertensives. Left ventricular hypertrophy is related to clinic measurements of blood pressure but also more closely related to ambulatory blood pressure. Both electrocardiographic and echocardiographic measures of left ventricular hypertrophy define a high risk population of hypertensives. Thus, in the Framingham Study (which initially only used electrocardiography) left ventricular hypertrophy was the strongest predictor of cardiovascular mortality in middle-aged adults. The risk of stroke or heart attack in hypertensive patients with echocardiographic left ventricular hypertrophy compared with patients without is increased fourfold (Fig. 10.13). Indeed, echocardiographically demonstrable increased left ventricular mass is a better predictor of risk than clinic blood pressure measurements.

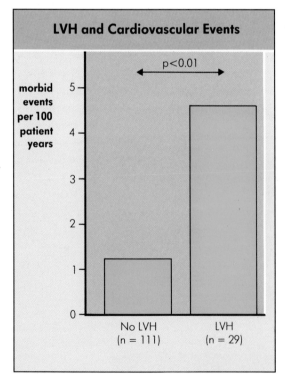

Fig. 10.13 Cardiovascular events occurring in 140 men with uncomplicated hypertension. The 29 patients with left ventricular hypertrophy showed a fourfold increase in events. (Modified from Casale et al. Ann Intern Med 1986; **105**:173–178.)

MECHANISMS AND RISK FACTORS IN LEFT VENTRICULAR HYPERTROPHY

The superior value of left ventricular hypertrophy as a risk predictor suggests that it is not simply acting as a marker of blood pressure elevation. One likely explanation is provided by the increased susceptibility of hearts, showing increased left ventricular mass, to ventricular arrhythmias. Another factor may be the increased myocardial oxygen demand of the hypertrophied ventricle, making it more susceptible to ischaemia.

There is considerable individual difference in the relationship between left ventricular hypertrophy and blood pressure elevation. It has, therefore, been suggested that several factors other than blood pressure may play a role in the pathogenesis of left ventricular hypertrophy. These are:

- genetic influences
- activity of the sympathetic nervous system
- the renin–angiotensin system (circulating and local cardiac systems).

These possible mechanisms have more than theoretical interest since, if they are important, one would anticipate differential effects of different hypertensive drugs on left ventricular mass. Some drugs, such as vasodilator antihypertensives which may increase cardiac work, have little effect on left ventricular mass. There is some evidence that diuretics have a lesser effect upon left ventricular mass than other antihypertensive agents. However, there are no adequately sized comparative trials to confirm this belief.

MANAGEMENT

The presence of left ventricular hypertrophy, associated with elevated blood pressure, is an indication for early and effective blood pressure control. The only satisfactory, generally available method for detecting it is, however, echocardiography and it is probably not justifiable to assess all hypertensive patients with echocardiography. Its major value is probably where there is an element of uncertainty about treatment, for example where a pressor response, to the act of blood pressure measurement, is suspected.

RENAL DISEASE

CLINICAL FEATURES

Renal disease is detected on screening patients, usually as a result of discovering proteinuria, elevated blood urea or serum creatinine. Where advanced hypertensive retinopathy is present, treatment of hypertension is a matter of urgency. Once blood pressure is controlled, patients can be investigated with kidney imaging and, if indicated, renal biopsy to establish whether hypertension is a result of or the cause of renal disease. Where advanced retinopathy is not present, proteinuria and/or renal failure are likely to be the result of renal vascular disease or renal parenchymatous disease. Imaging followed by, if necessary, renal biopsy are indicated. Rigorous blood pressure control is important in reducing the rate of decline of renal disease even where renal failure is not the result of hypertension.

RENAL FAILURE IN CARDIOVASCULAR DISEASE

Renal impairment is unusual in cardiovascular disease. Where the two coexist, the renal failure may be the result of cardiovascular disease or may be a risk factor in the development of cardiovascular disease.

Extensive Atheromatous Disease

This may reduce renal blood flow when the renal arteries are involved and, less commonly, may give rise to multiple cholesterol emboli in the kidney (Fig. 10.14).

Hypertensive Nephrosclerosis

Renal failure commonly occurs in accelerated (malignant) hypertension as a result of fibrinoid necrosis of the glomerular vessels (Fig. 10.15). Advanced renal failure is very rare in hypertensive patients where the disease has not entered an accelerated phase. However, the normal physiological decline in renal function with age is accelerated in the presence of uncontrolled hypertension. In the absence of advanced retinopathy, therefore, another cause for advanced renal failure should be sought in hypertension.

Antihypertensive Treatment

The fall in blood pressure produced by antihypertensive drugs may

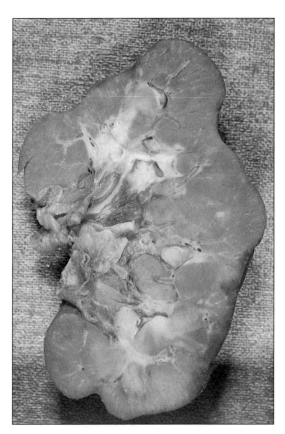

Fig. 10.14
Infarcts in the kidney secondary to multiple emboli. The scars can be shown by CT scanning (below).

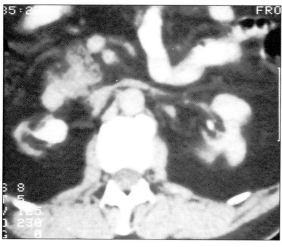

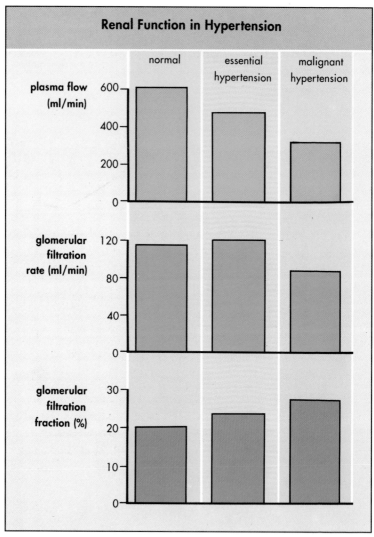

Fig. 10.15 Renal function in hypertension. Normally in essential hypertension without advanced retinopathy glomerular filtration rate is maintained despite a reduction in renal plasma flow. In malignant hypertension, however, glomerular filtration rate is reduced and renal failure may occur.

temporarily worsen renal impairment in malignant hypertension. This is a result of the fall in renal perfusion pressure. Sustained control of blood pressure, however, improves renal function in malignant hypertension as renal glomerular changes regress unless renal damage has already proceeded too far (Fig. 10.16).

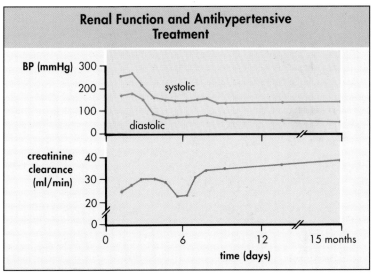

Fig. 10.16 Effect of antihypertensive treatment on blood pressure and renal function in a patient with malignant hypertension. A marked decrease in creatinine clearance occurred at the end of the first week. Renal function then improved progressively as renal hypertensive vascular damage was reversed.

ACE inhibitors may cause renal failure where renal blood flow is critically impaired as a result of bilateral or unilateral renal artery stenosis. Under these circumstances, glomerular filtration pressure is maintained by efferent glomerular arteriole vasoconstriction produced by angiotensin II. Removal of angiotensin II allows the efferent arteriole to dilate and glomerular filtration pressure falls. This effect may also be seen in patients treated for cardiac failure with ACE inhibitors (Fig. 10.17).

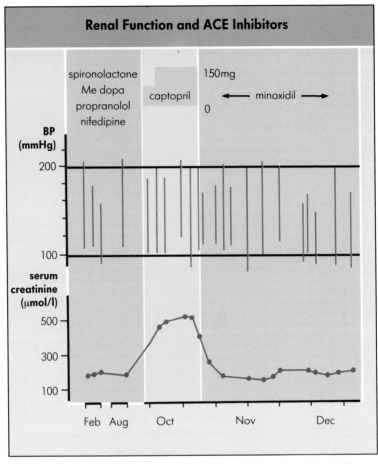

Fig. 10.17 Renal function, measured by serum creatinine, in a patient with bilateral renal artery stenosis, treated initially with a cocktail of drugs and then with captopril. Note that serum creatinine rose markedly when captopril was introduced. This decline of renal function was not the result of any fall in blood pressure. When captopril was stopped serum creatinine fell again.

RENAL DISEASE AS A RISK FACTOR

Primary renal disease increases the risk of morbidity or mortality from cardiovascular disease. Two factors have a role in this.

Hypertension

Elevated blood pressure is frequently observed in chronic renal disease, except for renal parenchymal disease associated with tubular damage where a sodium-losing state occurs. Hypertension is almost always observed at some stage in chronic glomerulonephritis and polycystic renal disease and frequently observed in chronic pyelonephritis. In the latter disease, there is a two-way relationship as pyelonephritis may give rise to an increased blood pressure but genetic predisposition to hypertension (shown by a positive family history) also predisposes to chronic pyelonephritis.

Metabolic Factors

Adverse circulating lipid changes are commonly seen in advanced renal disease, for example in patients on chronic dialysis. The death rate from cardiovascular disease is increased several-fold in such patients. Predisposition to vascular disease may be exacerbated by vascular calcification and insulin resistance, both of which are observed in chronic renal failure.

Medication as a Cardiovascular Risk Factor   11

Certain forms of medication increase risk factors (Fig. 11.1). Benefits of these drugs, therefore, have to be balanced against possible adverse effects.

Adverse Effects of some Medications	
Hypertension	**Lipids and other vascular risk factors**
Oestrogen-containing contraceptive pill	Oestrogen-containing contraceptive pill
Monoamine oxidase inhibitors and tyramine containing foods	Androgenic steroids
	Thiazide diuretics
Sympathomimetic amines in linctus	β-Blockers without sympathomimetic activity
Clonidine withdrawal	Erythropoietin
Nonsteroidal anti-inflammatory drugs	
Cyclosporin A	
Carbenoxolone	

Fig. 11.1 Commonly used drugs which have an adverse effect on cardiovascular risk factors.

OESTROGENS

In one large series of studies the cardiovascular death rate was found to be five times higher amongst women who took a high oestrogen-containing contraceptive pill (25.8 per 100,000 women years) compared to women who did not use the pill (5.5 per 100,000 women years). Causes of the excess mortality were myocardial infarction, thromboembolic disease and brain infarction.

The original high oestrogen-containing contraceptive pill produced elevations of blood pressure, adverse effects upon serum lipids, blood coagulation and glucose intolerance. As a result, the oestrogen content of the contraceptive pill has been reduced to 30μg per day or less. However, the effect on blood pressure may still be observed even at this dosage (Fig. 11.2). These adverse effects do not appear to occur with the progestogen only preparation.

Patients at risk of cardiovascular complications are those in whom other risk factors are present, i.e. women aged over 35 years, smokers, diabetics and women with hyperlipidaemia. The adverse effects of oestrogens on cardiovascular risk are probably not observed when they are

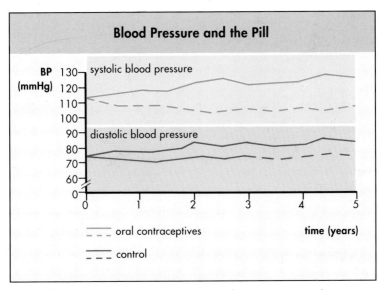

Fig. 11.2 Blood pressure changes in a group of women receiving the oestrogen-containing contraceptive pill. Both diastolic and systolic blood pressure rose gradually over five years of treatment.

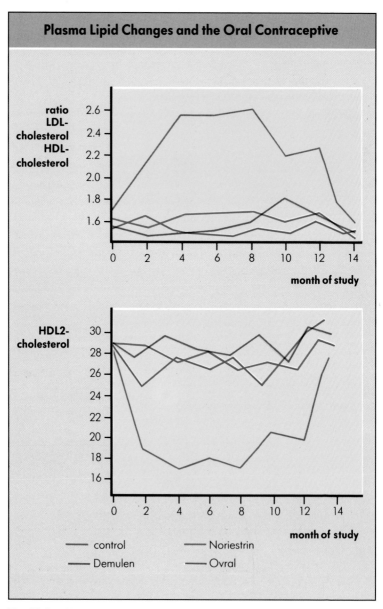

Fig. 11.3 Changes in plasma lipids with three oral contraceptives each containing 50µg ethinyloestradiol. The 'pill' (Ovral) with the most androgenic progestagen (dl-norgestrel) caused adverse changes. (Modified from La Rosa JC *Am J Obstet Gynecol* 1988; **158**:1621–1629.)

used as replacement therapy for menopausal symptoms and indeed in this situation blood pressure and risk of cardiovascular disease may be reduced.

It is essential to measure blood pressure in women prescribed the oestrogen-containing contraceptive pill, both before and during treatment. Oestrogen-containing contraceptive pills should be avoided in the higher risk patients mentioned previously and where hypertension develops in women receiving the oestrogen-containing contraceptive pill it should be stopped. Blood pressure may take several months or sometimes up to a year to decline to baseline levels after discontinuation. There is some anecdotal evidence for the development of permanent blood pressure elevation.

PROGESTAGENS

Retrospective studies have shown a relationship between the dose of progestagens in the contraceptive pill and the incidence of arterial disease. This seems to be related to the androgenic properties of the earlier synthesized progestagens. This gives rise to unfavourable changes in plasma lipids with a decrease in HDL2-cholesterol and an increase in LDL-cholesterol. More recently developed progestagens are less androgenic and do not have these adverse effects (Fig. 11.3).

OTHER DRUGS CAUSING HYPERTENSION

Ingestion of tyramine-containing cheeses by patients receiving monoamine oxidase inhibitors, sympathomimetic amines contained in some proprietary linctus preparations, which may be potentiated by post-ganglionic adrenergic blocking agents, and discontinuation of clonidine may all cause severe paroxysmal hypertension (Fig. 11.4).

Nonsteroidal anti-inflammatory drugs impair sodium and water excretion, particularly in elderly subjects. This may have a slight blood pressure elevating effect which is usually unimportant in normotensive individuals but may be important in patients receiving antihypertensive therapy. Administering anti-inflammatory drugs to such patients may cause loss of blood pressure control.

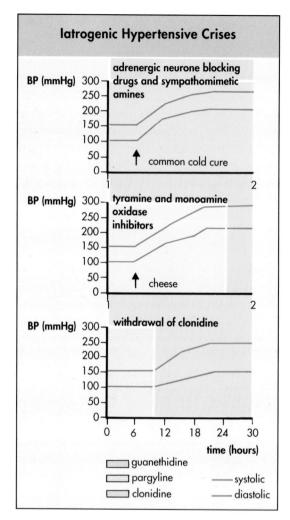

Fig. 11.4
Hypertensive crisis may be caused by medication. In each case paroxysmal hypertension was associated with evidence of sympathetic overactivity.

Carbenoxolone containing compounds used in the treatment of peptic ulceration may have the same effect. The immunosuppressive agent cyclosporin A used in the management of transplant patients frequently causes hypertension, although the mechanism is unknown.

MEDICATION AND OTHER CARDIOVASCULAR FACTORS

Thiazide diuretics cause a modest increase in total cholesterol, mainly reflecting an increase in LDL-cholesterol. This adverse effect can be largely avoided by a small dose of diuretic, e.g. bendrofluazide 2.5mg per day.

Adverse effects on serum lipids are also observed with β-adrenoceptor blockers (Fig. 11.5). These cause an increase in LDL-cholesterol and decrease in HDL-cholesterol with increased triglycerides. These effects are comparatively small, however, less evident with cardioselective agents and not observed with β-adrenoceptor blockers having intrinsic agonist activity, e.g. pindolol or celiprolol. ACE inhibitors have a neutral effect on lipids whilst α-blockers have a mildly beneficial effect.

Synthetic erythropoietin is widely used for the treatment of anaemia in dialysis patients. The increase in haematocrit which it produces is associated with both a rise in blood pressure and occasionally with brain infarction.

Metabolic Side Effects of some Antihypertensive Drugs

	β-Blockers	Diuretics	α-Blockers	ACE inhibitors	Ca antagonists
Blood glucose	↑?	↑	0	0	0?
Lipids					
HDL	↓ *	0	↑		
LDL	↑ *	↑	↓	0	0
TG	↑ *	↑	↓		
Serum urate	0	↑	0	0	0
Serum potassium		↓	0	↑	0?

*Less pronounced for selective β-blockers, and an opposite effect for β-blockers with marked intrinsic sympathomimetic activity

Fig. 11.5 Comparison between the metabolic side effects of different antihypertensive drugs. (Modifed from Brenner & Laragh, *Hypertension* (1990), Raven Press.)

175

Calculation of Risk 12

Long-term follow-up studies enable individual risk to be calculated from measured risk factors. The American Heart Association Risk Factor Charts are based upon the data from the Framingham Heart Study. Their importance lies both in identifying high risk patients who should be regarded as candidates for intensive treatment and for conveying to the clinician the relative importance of the risk factors discussed in this book.

Coronary Heart Disease Risk Factor Prediction Chart

1. Find Points for each Risk Factor

Age (if female)		Age (if male)		HDL-Cholesterol		Total-Cholesterol	
Age	Pts.	Age	Pts.	HDL-C	Pts.	Total-C	Pts.
30	−12	30	−2	25–26	7	139–151	−3
31	−11	31	−1	27–29	6	152–166	−2
32	−9	32–33	0	30–32	5	167–182	−1
33	−8	34	1	33–35	4	183–199	0
34	−6	35–36	2	36–38	3	200–219	1
35	−5	37–38	3	39–42	2	220–239	2
36	−4	39	4	43–46	1	240–262	3
37	−3	40–41	5	47–50	0	263–288	4
38	−2	42–43	6	51–55	−1	289–315	5
39	−1	44–45	7	56–60	−2	316–330	6
40	0	46–47	8	61–66	−3		
41	1	48–49	9	67–73	−4		
42–43	2	50–51	10	74–80	−5		
44	3	52–54	11	81–87	−6		
45–46	4	55–56	12	88–96	−7		
47–48	5	57–59	13				
49–50	6	60–61	14				
51–52	7	62–64	15				
53–55	8	65–67	16				
56–60	9	68–70	17				
61–67	10	71–73	18				
68–74	11	74	19				

Fig. 12.1   Coronary heart disease risk factor prediction chart.

176

Systolic Blood Pressure			Other	Pts.
SBP	Pts.			
98–104	-2		Cigarettes	4
105–112	-1		Diabetic male	3
113–120	0		Diabetic female	6
121–129	1		ECG-LVH	9
130–139	2			
140–149	3		0 pts for each NO	
150–160	4			
161–172	5			
173–185	6			

2. Sum Points for all Risk Factors

—— +	—— +	—— +	—— +	—— +	—— +	—— =	——
Age	HDL-C	Total-C	SBP	Smoker	Diabetes	ECG-LVH	Point Total

NOTE: Minus points subtract from total

3. Look up Risk Corresponding to Point Total

	Probability				Probability	
Pts.	5 Yr.	10 Yr.	Pts.		5 Yr.	10 Yr.
≤1	<1%	<2%	17		6%	13%
2	1%	2%	18		7%	14%
3	1%	2%	19		8%	16%
4	1%	2%	20		8%	18%
5	1%	3%	21		9%	19%
6	1%	3%	22		11%	21%
7	1%	4%	23		12%	23%
8	2%	4%	24		13%	25%
9	2%	5%	25		14%	27%
10	2%	6%	26		16%	29%
11	3%	6%	27		17%	31%
12	3%	7%	28		19%	33%
13	3%	8%	29		20%	36%
14	4%	9%	30		22%	38%
15	5%	10%	31		24%	40%
16	5%	12%	32		25%	42%

4. Compare to Average 10 Year Risk

	Probability	
Age	Women	Men
30–34	<1%	3%
35–39	<1%	5%
40–44	2%	6%
45–49	5%	10%
50–54	8%	14%
55–59	12%	16%
60–64	13%	21%
65–69	9%	30%
70–74	12%	24%

Stroke Risk Factor Prediction Chart

1. Find Points for each Risk Factor

Men

Age	SBP	HYP TR	Diabetes	Cigs	CVD	AF	LVH
54–56 = 0	95–105 = 0	No = 0	No = 0	No = 0	No = 0	No = 0	No = 0
57–59 = 1	106–116 = 1	Yes = 2	Yes = 2	Yes = 3	Yes = 3	Yes = 4	Yes = 6
60–62 = 2	117–126 = 2						
63–65 = 3	127–137 = 3						
66–68 = 4	138–148 = 4						
69–71 = 5	149–159 = 5						
72–74 = 6	160–170 = 6						
75–77 = 7	171–181 = 7						
78–80 = 8	182–191 = 8						
81–83 = 9	192–202 = 9						
84–86 = 10	203–213 = 10						

Women

Age	SBP	HYP TR	Diabetes	Cigs	CVD	AF	LVH
54–56 = 0	95–104 = 0	No = 0	No = 0	No = 0	No = 0	No = 0	No = 0
57–59 = 1	105–114 = 1	If Yes	Yes = 3	Yes = 3	Yes = 2	Yes = 6	Yes = 4
60–62 = 2	115–124 = 2	see					
63–65 = 3	125–134 = 3	below					
66–68 = 4	135–144 = 4						
69–71 = 5	145–154 = 5						
72–74 = 6	155–164 = 6						
75–77 = 7	165–174 = 7						
78–80 = 8	175–184 = 8						
81–83 = 9	185–194 = 9						
84–86 = 10	195–204 = 10						

If currently under antihypertensive therapy add the following points depending on SBP level

SBP	95–104	105–114	115–124	125–134	135–144	145–154
Points	6	5	5	4	3	3

SBP	155–164	165–174	175–184	185–194	195–204
Points	2	1	1	0	0

Key for symbols:

SBP	– Systolic blood pressure
HYP TR	– Under antihypertensive therapy?
Diabetes	– History of diabetes?
Cigs	– Smokes cigarettes?
CVD	– History of myocardial infarction, angina pectoris, coronary insufficiency, intermittent claudication or congestive heart failure?
AF	– History of atrial fibrillation?
LVH	– Left ventricular hypertrophy on ECG?

Fig. 12.2 Stroke risk factor prediction chart. Only risk factors which were shown to be of importance are included in these charts. Systolic blood pressure

2. Sum Points for all Risk Factors

___	+	___	+	___	+	___	+	___	+	___	+	___	+	___	=	___
Age		SBP		HYP TR		Diabetes		Cigs		CVD		AF		LVH		Point Total

3. Look up Risk Corresponding to Point Total

	Probability Men		**Probability Women**
Pts.	10 Yr.	Pts.	10 Yr.
1	2.6%	1	1.1%
2	3.0%	2	1.3%
3	3.5%	3	1.6%
4	4.0%	4	2.0%
5	4.7%	5	2.4%
6	5.4%	6	2.9%
7	6.3%	7	3.5%
8	7.3%	8	4.3%
9	8.4%	9	5.2%
10	9.7%	10	6.3%
11	11.2%	11	7.6%
12	12.9%	12	9.2%
13	14.8%	13	11.1%
14	17.0%	14	13.3%
15	19.5%	15	16.0%
16	22.4%	16	19.1%
17	25.5%	17	22.8%
18	29.0%	18	27.0%
19	32.9%	19	31.9%
20	37.1%	20	37.3%
21	41.7%	21	43.4%
22	46.6%	22	50.0%
23	51.8%	23	57.0%
24	57.3%	24	64.2%
25	62.8%	25	71.4%
26	68.4%	26	78.2%
27	73.8%	27	84.4%
28	79.0%		
29	83.7%		
30	87.9%		

4. Compare to Average 10 Year Risk

		Probability	
Age	Men	Age	Women
55–59	5.9%	55–59	3.0%
60–64	7.8%	60–64	4.7%
65–69	11.0%	65–69	7.2%
70–74	13.7%	70–74	10.9%
75–79	18.0%	75–79	15.5%
80–84	22.3%	80–84	23.9%

alone is presented, as the addition of diastolic blood pressure to the information provided by a knowledge of systolic blood pressure was not significant.

INDEX

182

183